The Lighthouse Principle

Why Medical Errors Occur — And How to Prevent Them

William H. Light, M.D.

Published by The Lighthouse Watchman Press

ISBN 979-8-9971632-0-4 (paperback)

First Edition, 2026

Contents

FOREWORD 1

Part I 3
The Case for Thinking Slowly

PART I — CHAPTER 1 5
Premature Closure — *The Lighthouse Principle*

PART I — CHAPTER 2 9
Anchoring Bias — *The First Label*

PART I — CHAPTER 3 14
Confirmation Bias — *What You Came In Looking For*

PART I — CHAPTER 4 19
Search Satisfaction — *The Answer That Wasn't Enough*

PART I — CHAPTER 5 24
Framing Effect — *The Story You Inherit*

PART I — CHAPTER 6 28
Availability Bias — *The Last Case*

PART I — CHAPTER 7 33
Representative Bias — *The Rash That Never Came*

PART I — CHAPTER 8 37
Overconfidence Bias — *The Confident Mind*

PART I — CHAPTER 9 42
Diagnosis Momentum — *The Diagnosis That Traveled*

PART I — CHAPTER 10 48
Time Pressure Bias — *The Shortcut They Purchased*

PART I — CHAPTER 11 55
Outcome Bias — *The Question That Felt Answered*

PART I — CHAPTER 12 61
Hindsight Bias — *The Obvious Answer*

Part II 68
When Thinking Fails

PART II — CHAPTER 1 70
Narrative Coherence Bias — *The Story That Fit Too Well*

PART II — CHAPTER 2 75
Narrative Compression — *The Interrupted Story*

PART II — CHAPTER 3 80
Cognitive Dissonance — *The Patient Who Would Not Make Sense*

PART II — CHAPTER 4 85
Authority Bias — *The Voice That Ends the Discussion*

PART II — CHAPTER 5 90
Groupthink — *The Diagnosis Everyone Agreed On*

PART II — CHAPTER 6 96
Cognitive Ease — *The Shortcut Everyone Took*

PART II — CHAPTER 7 101
Normalization of Deviance — *The Exception Everyone Stopped Noticing*

PART II — CHAPTER 8 106
Protocol Fixation — *The Patient Who Did Not Fit the Protocol*

PART II — CHAPTER 9 112
Moral Disengagement — *The Case That Felt Smaller*

PART II — CHAPTER 10 118
Diffusion of Responsibility — *The Decision No One Owned*

PART II — CHAPTER 11 124
What Experience Forgets — *The Patient Nobody Would Examine*

PART II — CHAPTER 12 129
The Discipline of Pause — *What Maya Learns to Hold*

Part III 138
What We Leave Behind

PART III — CHAPTER 1 140
What Survives the Teacher — *Noah's First Night*

PART III — CHAPTER 2 143
The Wrong Hands — *What Elias Would Not Sign Off On*

PART III — CHAPTER 3 148
When Criteria Are Not Enough — *Before I Go Home*

PART III — CHAPTER 4 154
The Question You Inherit — *"What Would Make This Not What I Think It Is."*

PART III — CHAPTER 5 157
Borrowed Confidence — *Often Wrong, Never in Doubt*

PART III — CHAPTER 6 161
The Limits of the Method — *When the Disease Asks the Question*

PART III — CHAPTER 7 165
What the Junior Sees First — *The Pattern Across the Rooms*

PART III — CHAPTER 8 171
The Cost of Being Right — *What Silence Costs the Room*

PART III — CHAPTER 9 175
When the Lines Cross — *Whose Patient Is She*

PART III — CHAPTER 10 179
What the Bed Conceals — *The View from the Chair*

PART III — CHAPTER 11 183
The Discovery — *The Teacher Becomes the Patient*

PART III — CHAPTER 12 189
The Habit That Outlives the Room — *What Remains*

AFTERWORD 193

Foreword

I became chief resident in 1985.

I did not know then what I know now about how teaching works. I knew how to present a case cleanly. I knew how to run a differential. I knew how to move a busy service through a difficult morning without losing anyone. I thought that was most of what teaching required — clarity, efficiency, the right answer arrived at quickly enough to model for the people watching.

I was wrong about that. What I did not know in 1985 was that the residents and students rotating through my service were not primarily learning from what I said. They were learning from what I did when I didn't know the answer. They were learning from whether I sat down or stayed standing. They were learning from whether I went back to a room after rounds or kept moving. They were learning from the questions I asked out loud and the ones I kept to myself, from whether I said I don't know yet in front of a team or protected everyone — including myself — from that discomfort.

Throughout four decades of internal medicine, I tutored medical students, residents, nurse practitioners, and medical assistants. I watched some of them become extraordinary clinicians and I watched others become fast ones, and I slowly learned to tell the difference early. It was never the fund of knowledge. It was never the board scores. It was whether they had acquired, from someone, somewhere, the habit of staying in the question a moment longer than the room required. That habit is almost never taught deliberately. It is absorbed — from a teacher who models it often enough that the student stops noticing they are learning it at all. This book is my attempt to write that absorption down.

The people in these pages are fictional. The errors are not. The cases are real, a mixture of what I have experienced and shared with my fellow clinicians over years of medical practice. Every cognitive trap in this book I have watched happen, and many of them I have committed myself — some of them more than once, a few of them in ways I still think about. The cases have been altered, combined, and relocated until no patient could recognize themselves, but the reasoning failures are rendered exactly as they occur in real hospitals, because softening them would defeat the purpose of the book.

The question at the center of these chapters is simple. What would make this not what I think it is. If you take nothing else from this book, take that. Ask it before the story closes. Ask it especially when the story feels finished, because that feeling is the most dangerous moment in medicine.

Everything else in these pages is an illustration of what happens when someone asks it — and what it costs when no one does.

William H. Light, M.D.

Part I

The Case for Thinking Slowly

Medicine rewards answers. Training reinforces them, rounds demand them, charts memorialize them. But patients rarely arrive with answers. They arrive with fragments, contradictions, stories that do not behave.

Most diagnostic errors do not occur because clinicians lack knowledge. They occur because thinking stops too soon. This book is not about rare diseases. It is about common mistakes — about the moment when a diagnosis feels right, when the story seems to fit, when the urge to stop thinking becomes irresistible. That moment is critical.

The cases in this book are not puzzles to be solved. They are stories to be listened to. Each chapter explores a single cognitive trap that shapes clinical reasoning, and each case unfolds the way real cases do — messy, incomplete, fragmented, uncooperative. There are no algorithms here, no shortcuts, no guarantees. Only a method: a way of noticing, a way of pausing, a way of asking better questions.

The most important of those questions is simple. What does not belong. Learn to ask it honestly and you will miss fewer diagnoses and make fewer assumptions. Not because you know more. Because you stop erasing too quickly.

PART I — CHAPTER 1

Premature Closure

The Lighthouse Principle

When the story does not fit, widen the lens.
The first answer is rarely the right one.
The danger is not what you do not know.
It is what you stop looking for.

Sunlight cut through the tall windows of Westside Hospital. July first. The day medicine rearranged itself. Students became interns, interns became residents, and residents stepped closer to the edge where independence met accountability.

At the center of the room stood Dr. Elara Holt. New chief resident. Posture precise, voice steady. Today mattered.

"For the next two months," she said, "you will be working under Dr. Henry Lighthouse."

A few of the interns glanced at each other.

"He is not known for speed. He is known for accuracy." She paused. "When he first arrived here, a group of residents tried to stump him with what they pretended was a straightforward cellulitis case. They simplified the story. They hid the details." Her voice lowered. "He examined the patient once and said: Observe the crepitus under the skin. Pallor in the nail beds. Faint yellowing of the conjunctiva. Gas-forming bacteria. Hemolysis. Jaundice. This is Clostridium perfringens, he stated. Likely from shoveling peat moss."

She hesitated.

"Then he added: Those nodules along the forearm. Beaded. Linear. Sporothrix. He is a rose gardener."

Silence.

"None of them understood what he said that day. That is not the lesson — the lesson is that he was looking at a man, and they were looking for an answer. He came here from the East Coast, an outsider with a reputation for excellence. He has proven that and more." She let that sit. "So, if any of you decide to challenge him, remember — a near miss is still a miss."

The door opened. Dr. Henry Lighthouse entered without urgency. White coat pressed, eyes alert. He surveyed the room once.

"Good morning. Let us begin."

The conference room hummed softly. Lighthouse stood at the whiteboard, hands behind his back.

"Elias," he said. "You have the new admission."

Intern Elias Ward cleared his throat. It was his first call night. He had not slept.

"Sixty-eight-year-old man. One week history of cough and fever. Chest X-ray shows right lower lobe pneumonia." He glanced at his notes. "Started on antibiotics overnight. Temperature down this morning." He looked up. "Most likely community-acquired pneumonia."

The room nodded. Lighthouse said nothing.

Elias continued. "He also reports fatigue, night sweats, and a ten-pound weight loss."

Lighthouse paused, then he looked at him. "His wife is in the room," he said. "She has been there all night. Suppose she asks you what is wrong with her husband. What do you tell her."

Elias hesitated. "That he has pneumonia. An infection in the lung. That the antibiotics are working and his fever is coming down."

"And when she asks you why he has lost ten pounds."

The room went quiet.

"One week of cough is pneumonia," Lighthouse said. "Ten pounds and night sweats is a story about the time before the cough. You have answered the first question. She is asking the second one."

Lighthouse studied the board. Then he quietly erased the word pneumonia. Just that word, nothing else. No explanation.

"What else explains fatigue, night sweats, and weight loss," he said.

Silence. Elias felt the word forming but did not say it. Malignancy.

Dr. Holt answered. "Chronic infection. Autoimmune disease. Tuberculosis. Malignancy."

"Good," Lighthouse said. "Let us see him."

At the bedside, Mr. Carter looked exhausted.

"When did the fatigue begin," Lighthouse asked.

"About three months ago," the patient said. "Thought it was age."

Lighthouse listened to the lungs. Crackles on the right. The pneumonia was real. He felt the abdomen. He paused.

"The spleen is enlarged," he said. Not as a revelation. As the finding that changed everything.

In the hallway, Lighthouse turned to him.

"The pneumonia is real," he said. "It is not the complete diagnosis." He paused. "You had the findings. Fatigue. Night sweats. Weight loss. An enlarged spleen. You explained all of it with the infection and stopped." He turned to Elias. "When the story does not fit," he said, "widen the lens."

He turned and walked back toward the workroom.

The workup told the rest of it. Imaging. A bone marrow biopsy. Lymphoma. Early stage. Treatable. The pneumonia had been real. Treating it had been correct. It had also been incomplete.

That night, Elias wrote in his notebook.

When the story does not fit,
widen the lens.

He closed the book.

Clinical Reflection

Premature closure is rarely a wrong answer. It is a real one, found early, that stops the search — a true finding earns a trust that spreads, absorbing even the symptoms it cannot explain. Nothing feels missing, because something true has been found. That is what makes it the most common error in medicine and the hardest to feel: the pneumonia is real, the fracture is real, the positive test is real, and each one quietly closes the door on everything it does not account for. The discipline is easy to name and easy to forget at two in the morning: once the first answer arrives, ask what it does not explain. If the answer is something — a weight loss, a night sweat, an edge you can barely feel beneath the ribs — do not file it away. Let it reopen the case. The first diagnosis is not the enemy. Letting it be the last one is. Erase the answer that is blocking the view, and look again.

PART I — CHAPTER 2

Anchoring Bias

The First Label

The first label is the most dangerous.
It clings.
And it makes everything after it
bend toward it.

Elias was moving fast. The hallway was busy. Mid-morning. The kind of Tuesday that accumulates without warning. Charts stacking. Pagers going. The ward finding its rhythm.

He was three steps past the room when Lighthouse stopped. Not urgently. Not dramatically. He simply stopped.

Elias turned.

Lighthouse was looking through the open doorway. Not at the chart on the door. Not at the monitor visible from the hall. At the patient.

She was sitting upright in bed. Middle aged. Small. Neat. The kind of woman who apologized for taking up space. She was breathing carefully. Not obviously struggling.

But her face was wrong.

It was the face of a woman who had been given an explanation that did not match what she was experiencing. Bewildered. Not frightened. A woman who had been told what was wrong with her and knew, without knowing how, that it was incorrect.

Lighthouse recognized her. From clinic. From past years of quiet appointments. From the way she sat in a chair and composed herself.

He went in.

She looked up when he entered. Something shifted in her face. Not relief exactly. Something quieter. Recognition — the recognition of a patient who has been waiting for the right person to walk through the door.

"Tell me what's been happening," Lighthouse said. He pulled up a chair. Sat beside her.

She spoke carefully. "They say it's asthma," she said. "But I don't understand it. I've never had asthma. I don't smoke. I've never had allergies. Not once in my life." She looked at her hands. "I just don't understand how this happened. At sixty-two. Out of nowhere."

At the bedside, Elias reviewed the chart quietly.

The notes were consistent. Confident. Each one copied the one before.

Wheezing. Asthma. Inhaler prescribed.

The diagnosis had arrived before she did. Attached to her name. Traveling with her from clinic to hospital. No one had questioned it. Why would they. She wheezed. She had no smoking history. COPD was excluded. Asthma fit.

The label had done what labels do. It had made the thinking feel finished.

Lighthouse examined her without hurry. Listened to the lungs. Wheezing, faint, bilateral. That fit the label. He moved the stethoscope. Listened to the heart.

Then he stopped.

Elias watched him. The pause was different from the others. Longer. More still.

Lighthouse repositioned. Leaned slightly forward. Then straightened.

"Can you lean forward for me," he asked.

She did.

He listened again. Left sternal border. Apex. Right upper sternal border. Then he removed the stethoscope from his ears. He did not speak immediately. He handed Elias his stethoscope — his signature double-tube Sprague-Rappaport, heavy as a stone in the hand, chrome faded at the edges from forty plus years of pockets.

Not as instruction. Not as theater. Simply as an invitation.

Elias took it. Adjusted the earpieces. Leaned forward the way Lighthouse had.

The wheezing was there. He heard it first, the way you always hear what you expect. He moved the diaphragm. Repositioned.

And then — beneath the wheeze, beneath the noise of a room that had already decided what it was hearing — something else. Quiet, but harsh. A murmur that did not announce itself.

He straightened. Removed the stethoscope. Carefully handed it back to Lighthouse.

Lighthouse was quiet. He was watching him.

"Has anyone listened carefully to your heart," Lighthouse asked her.

She thought. "I don't think so," she said. "They always listened to my breathing."

"Of course they did," Lighthouse said. Quietly. Without judgment.

In the hallway, Lighthouse stopped.

"What would make this not asthma," he said.

Elias felt the question land differently than he expected — less a challenge than a door left open.

"If the wheezing was caused by upper airway obstruction, GERD, respiratory infection, or had a cardiac source," he said slowly. "And if she had never actually responded to the inhalers."

Lighthouse studied him. "Had she," he asked.

Elias was quiet a moment. "No one asked," he said.

Lighthouse nodded. "What did you hear," he said.

Elias hesitated. "A murmur. Systolic. Harsh but faint. Loudest at the right upper sternal border. Radiating toward the neck."

He let the finding sit there.

"Aortic stenosis."

The word arrived in a way he had not expected — not a diagnosis so much as an answer to a question that had been sitting unanswered in a woman's face.

"The wheezing is real," Lighthouse said. "Cardiac asthma — but that is not asthma at all. The wheeze is not bronchospasm. It comes from a heart that cannot keep up. And no one asked the one question that would have said so."

Elias thought of the chart. The notes copied forward. The inhalers prescribed. The label traveling with her from appointment to appointment.

"That is why the inhalers didn't help," he said.

"They didn't hurt either. Not enough to raise a flag. She compensated. She adapted."

Elias looked back through the doorway. She was sitting in the same position. Upright. Careful. Waiting.

"She knew something was wrong," Elias said.

"Yes," Lighthouse said. "She just didn't know she was allowed to say so."

Lighthouse went back in. He pulled the chair up again and sat.

"I want to tell you what I heard," he said.

She folded her hands and waited.

"There is a valve in your heart. The aortic valve. It functions as a door that blood passes through on its way out to the body. It has narrowed. It happens slowly, over years — calcium builds on the valve, and it stiffens, and it opens a little less each year. Your heart has been pushing against it for a long time. When blood cannot leave the heart easily, it backs up into the lungs. That is the wheezing. The sound is real." He paused. "But it is not asthma. It never was."

She was quiet. "So, I didn't become a different person at sixty-two."

"No," Lighthouse said. "You have been the same person all along. The valve was simply closing so slowly that you learned to live with it. Most people would have complained years ago. You adapted instead."

"Can it be fixed."

"The valve can be replaced. We will do an echocardiogram, a picture of your heart with ultrasound, this afternoon to be certain. But I believe that is what we will find."

Something in her face changed — not relief at the news, which was, after all, a diagnosis of a failing heart valve. And she was facing heart surgery. Relief at the explanation. At a story that finally matched her life.

The echocardiogram returned that afternoon. Severe aortic stenosis. Valve area critically reduced. Gradient significantly elevated.

Cardiac surgery was consulted. The surgery went well. Three weeks later she walked out of the hospital without stopping to apologize to anyone for the space she took up.

That evening Lighthouse stopped in the doorway of the workroom.

"The murmur was there," he said. Elias looked up. "Every visit. Waiting to be heard by someone who wasn't already listening for something else." He paused. "The label didn't cause the murmur to disappear. It caused the mind to stop looking for it."

Elias nodded. He thought of the moment in the room. The stethoscope passed without a word. The sound beneath the sound he was already listening for.

"What made you go in," he asked.

Lighthouse considered the question. "Her face," he said.

He did not elaborate.

That night Elias wrote in his notebook.

The patient often knows before we do.
The finding was there. I was listening for something else.

Clinical Reflection

Anchoring needs no wrong diagnosis — only a label applied early enough to shape everything after it. It is usually plausible, usually backed by something real, which is what lets it travel from note to note, each encounter adding weight without adding examination. The finding that would undo it is seldom hidden; it is simply never sought, because no one inside the frame has a reason to look. The antidote is not suspicion. It is asking, before the exam begins, what would make this not the diagnosis already attached to the patient — then entering as if hearing the story for the first time.

PART I — CHAPTER 3

Confirmation Bias

What You Came In Looking For

The moment medicine becomes most vulnerable
is when the diagnosis feels settled.
Not because you found the answer.
But because you stopped looking for another one.

The triage note was two words. Under the caption 'Chief Complaint' were the words 'Sore Throat.' That was all it took. Two words written by a nurse doing her job efficiently in a department moving too fast to pause over a retired schoolteacher with a sore throat. Two words that became a frame. A lens. A filter through which everything that followed was seen and sorted and made to fit.

The clinician read them before entering the room. That mattered.

She was sixty-five years old. Neat. Quiet. She had spent forty years making sure other people were comfortable before attending to herself. She was lying down. Not sitting on the edge of the table. Not leaning forward. On her back. Still.

He noted this briefly. He asked her to sit up. She had to use her elbows to push herself up. He noticed this as well. Then he moved to examine her throat.

The posterior pharynx was mildly erythematous. Not dramatically — no exudate, no swelling — but red enough. Red enough to confirm what the triage note had already suggested. Red enough to allow the examination to feel complete.

The temperature was one hundred, slightly elevated. The white count was ten point five, again mildly elevated. Nonspecific. Strep screen negative. Consistent with early viral illness.

She reported throat discomfort. Mild. Hard to localize exactly. "Sometimes it feels more like pressure," she said.

He nodded. Wrote something down.

Then she said something else. Quietly. Almost as a correction to herself.

"My throat isn't sore, exactly," she said. "It just — hurts. And it does not hurt when I swallow."

He looked up briefly. He was already writing the discharge instructions.

Viral syndrome, the note read. Possible early pharyngitis.

The nurse handed her the discharge instructions. Rest. Fluids. Follow up if worsening.

She thanked her. Without complaint. Without demand. She went home.

She came back that night.

Elias was there when the doors opened. She arrived by ambulance this time. Diaphoretic. Hypotensive. Clutching her chest with both hands. The EKG told the truth immediately. Massive anterior ST elevation — tombstone waves across the precordium. An LAD occlusion announcing itself with the brutality of a vessel that has been closing all day and has finally finished.

The cath lab was activated. The service did not stop. There were other patients. Other charts. Other decisions that could not wait. Elias moved through the rest of the night the way interns do. Forward. Without pause.

Later, near the end of his shift, he stopped by the cardiology unit. Not because it was required. Because something pulled him. The cardiologist was finishing his note. "Massive anterior MI," he said without looking up. "LAD occlusion. Successful angioplasty. She's stable. For now." He paused. "Close thing."

Elias did not know her name yet. He did not know she had been here that morning. He only knew that someone had almost not made it, and that the cardiologist's voice carried the flatness of a physician who had seen how close it was and was not yet done with it.

The next morning Lighthouse called a meeting. Small. Quiet. The kind that does not appear on any schedule. Elias was there. The clinician who had seen her that morning sat at the end of the table with the stillness of someone who had not slept.

Lighthouse did not begin with the outcome. He began with the triage note. He wrote it on the whiteboard. Chief Complaint: Sore Throat. Then he turned.

"Walk me through the visit," he said. Not unkindly. With the specific attention of someone who needed to understand exactly where the thinking had gone.

He spoke carefully. The triage note. The erythema. The mild temperature. The mild white count. The discharge. Lighthouse listened without interrupting.

When he finished the room was quiet. Elias looked at the whiteboard. He thought of a question. He asked it before he decided to.

"What would make this not viral pharyngitis," he said.

The room turned toward him. He had not meant it as a challenge. He meant it the way he was beginning to understand it needed to be meant — as the first question. Not the last one.

Lighthouse watched him. Then turned back to the whiteboard.

"Yes," he said. "Exactly that."

He wrote one question beneath the triage note. Why was she lying down.

"She said she was tired."

"And," Lighthouse said.

A long pause. "I thought it fit. With a viral illness."

Lighthouse nodded. He did not press harder. "A patient with a sore throat sits up," he said. "They are uncomfortable. They want water. They lean forward. A patient lying flat on a table is telling you something their chief complaint has not said yet.

"You walked in looking for a sore throat," he said. "And you found one. Mild erythema. Which should have been the beginning of a question." He paused. "Not the end of one."

Beneath 'Why was she lying down' he wrote two more lines. 'Throat pain as anginal equivalent. Stuttering infarction.'

"The heart has no vocabulary for its own pain. Its signal enters the spinal cord alongside the nerves of the arm, the back, and the epigastrium — and the brain assigns the ache to the neighbor it knows better. Jaw. Arm. Back. Epigastrium." He paused. "And Throat."

He looked at the clinician. "What was her risk profile," he asked.

"Sixty-five-year-old woman," he said. "Hypertension. Hyperlipidemia. Family history of cardiac disease. Postmenopausal."

"The risk factors were in the chart," Lighthouse said. "Available to anyone who looked before deciding what they were looking for." He set down the marker. "And she said it directly. My throat isn't sore, exactly. It just hurts. And it does not hurt to swallow. She was distinguishing between the two. Offering the disconfirming detail herself." He paused. "It was filed under viral syndrome and pharyngitis."

He turned to the clinician. "Confirmation bias does not require laziness," he said. "It requires only a diagnosis that feels final before the patient has finished speaking."

The clinician nodded once. Slowly. The nod of someone absorbing something they will carry for the rest of their career.

After the others left Elias stood at the whiteboard. He thought of the triage note. He thought of the woman lying flat. He thought honestly about what he would have done if he had walked into that room first. He would have turned to her throat. He would have seen the erythema and felt the frame close around him. He knew that without any doubt.

The question he had asked that morning in the meeting — what would make this not viral pharyngitis — he would not have asked it either. Not then.

But he had asked it this morning. In a room where it was too late to matter for her.

He was not yet sure what that meant.

Lighthouse stood beside him. "She survived," Elias said.

"Yes," Lighthouse said.

"Will she be all right."

"Her heart has been changed," Lighthouse said. "How much we will learn over time." He paused. "She is a retired schoolteacher," he said. "She did know something was wrong. She trusted that the person in the white coat knew more than she did about what her body was saying." He turned. "Our job is to be worthy of that assumption."

Elias nodded. He thought of her lying flat on the table. Still. Quiet. Waiting for someone to ask the right question. Offering the answer herself, once, and watching it be filed away.

That night he wrote in his notebook.

She corrected her own story.
He had already decided what that meant.
I asked the question today. Too late.
In time, I hope, for the next one.

Clinical Reflection

Confirmation bias begins with a label that arrives before the clinician does, and a finding that confirms it — usually real, usually weak, enough only to let an exam that started with an answer feel finished. The disconfirming evidence is there too: visible from the doorway, or spoken once in the patient's own quiet correction. A frame already closed absorbs both without registering either. So enter without a conclusion already forming, look at the whole patient before the part they came in for, and when a patient corrects their own complaint, stop. That moment is not a detail. It is the diagnosis asking to be reconsidered.

PART I — CHAPTER 4

Search Satisfaction

The Answer That Wasn't Enough

Finding something
is not the same as finding everything.
The mind declares victory too soon.
And the real answer waits in the question
nobody thought to ask.

The consult came at eleven-fifteen. Not urgent enough for a page. Urgent enough that the cardiology fellow called directly.

"We've got a sixty-year-old male," he said. "Post cath. Still hypotensive. We've done everything."

Elias heard the exhaustion in the fellow's voice. Not defeat. The frustration of a thorough workup that had produced an insufficient answer.

"What did the cath show," Elias asked.

"Moderate CAD. Two vessel disease. Non-obstructive. Nothing that should be doing this to his pressure." A pause. "Echo beforehand showed an EF of forty percent. Scarring in the inferior wall. Consistent with a prior silent event. So we know we have a sick heart. Real disease. Documented. And a man who has been on pressors for six hours and still isn't responding the way he should."

"The team feels this is ischemic cardiomyopathy," he said. "But something isn't right. I need a new set of eyes on this. Can you take a look?"

Elias picked up his pen. "I'll come down," he said.

The chart was thick. Elias read it carefully before entering the room.

The story was orderly. Well documented. The kind of workup that reflects genuine effort and genuine intelligence. Sixty years old. Hypertension. Hyperlipidemia. Strong family history of coronary disease. Presented hypotensive. A cardiac risk profile that justified every decision the cardiology team had made.

The echo had been the right call — an abnormal finding that demanded explanation. The cath had followed logically. Everything it turned up was real and documented: genuine disease, a prior event nobody had known about.

Ischemic cardiomyopathy.

The story had assembled itself from genuine findings into something that looked, from inside the cardiology workup, exactly like an answer. A sick heart. Documented disease. A mechanism for hypotension.

The search had felt complete. It was not.

Elias turned the pages.

Something caught his eye.

Sodium one twenty-six.

He stopped. Read the note attached to it. Hyponatremia likely dilutional in setting of aggressive fluid resuscitation. He sat with that. It was possible. Plausible. The kind of explanation that arrives when a finding needs to be filed away so the main story can continue.

Then he turned back to the admission labs.

Sodium one twenty-four on arrival. Before the fluids. Before the echo. Before the cath. Before any of the careful, well-reasoned cardiology workup that had produced a coherent story about a sick heart and still hadn't explained why this man's blood pressure refused to move.

He set down the chart.

The patient was a solidly built man who looked smaller than his history suggested. Lying still. Blood pressure eighty-eight systolic on two pressors. His face carrying the gray color of a body running out of reserves.

Elias pulled up a chair. Sat.

"Tell me about yourself," he said. Not: tell me about your symptoms. Not: walk me through what happened. Tell me about yourself.

The man looked at him. Something shifted slightly in his face. "What do you want to know," he said.

"Whatever feels important," Elias said.

A pause.

The man spoke slowly. Retired engineer. Lived alone since his wife passed. Had been seeing his doctor for joint pain. Hands mostly. Some mornings worse than others.

"They thought it might be arthritis," he said. "Started me on something for it."

Elias kept his face still. "What did they start you on," he said.

The man hesitated — deciding whether to admit the thing he had been holding back.

"Prednisone," he said. He did not look at Elias when he said it.

"How long ago," Elias asked.

"About six weeks."

"And are you still taking it."

Another pause. Longer.

"I stopped," the man said. His voice was careful. Measured. The voice of a man who had made a decision he wasn't proud of and had been waiting all day for someone to find it. "About a week ago."

"Can I ask why," Elias said.

The man studied his hands. "The weight," he said. "I put on eight pounds in a month. My face looked different." He paused. "I didn't tell my doctor. I just stopped." He finally looked up. "I should have told someone. I know that now."

Elias sat with what he had just been given.

The hyponatremia. The refractory hypotension. Prednisone stopped abruptly after six weeks. A body that had forgotten how to make its own cortisol and had been asked to manage a crisis without it.

The answer came together all at once — everything scattered finding its arrangement.

Adrenal crisis.

He called the attending. "I think this is adrenal insufficiency," he said. "Prednisone stopped abruptly a week ago. Hyponatremia present on admission before fluids. Refractory hypotension despite adequate resuscitation and a cardiac explanation that accounts for some of his dysfunction but not the severity of what we're seeing. I want to give him a stress dose of hydrocortisone."

A pause on the other end. "Go ahead," the attending said.

The nurse hung the hydrocortisone at twelve forty-seven. Elias stayed.

At one-fifteen the systolic touched ninety-four. At one-thirty it was one hundred and two. By two a.m. the first pressor had been weaned.

The man was watching the monitor too. "Is it working," he asked.

"Yes," Elias said.

The man exhaled — a long slow release of something he had been holding since long before he arrived at the hospital.

"I should have told my doctor," he said again.

"You told me," Elias said.

The man nodded. He closed his eyes. His color was already different.

The next morning Lighthouse found Elias at the nursing station and sat down beside him.

"Walk me through it," he said.

Elias did. The consult. The thick chart. The echo and the cath, and the internally consistent cardiology story built from real findings that genuinely fit together. The sodium that didn't fit the explanation given for it. The chair pulled up beside the bed. The question that wasn't about symptoms. The prednisone.

Lighthouse listened without interrupting.

"What made you notice the sodium," he said.

"It was low before the fluids," Elias said. "Before the echo. Before any of the cardiology workup. The explanation in the chart didn't hold once I looked at the timeline." He paused. "And something about the whole picture felt wrong. A reduced EF with moderate disease explains some dysfunction. It doesn't explain a man who won't come off pressors despite appropriate resuscitation."

Lighthouse considered that. "The cardiology team did their job," he said. "The echo was right. The cath was right. The moderate CAD was real. The reduced EF was real." He paused. "But a real finding is not always the right answer. It is sometimes just enough of an answer to make everyone stop looking."

He watched Elias. "Everyone else accepted the explanation. You didn't."

Elias nodded. "He was embarrassed," he said. "He'd stopped the prednisone without telling anyone."

Lighthouse considered this. "Patients protect us from information they think will disappoint us," he said. "Your job is to make the room safe enough that they don't have to." He stood. "You did that last night," he said, and left without elaborating.

That night Elias wrote in his notebook.

A real finding is not always the right answer.

Sometimes it is just enough to make everyone stop looking.

Make the room safe enough.

The answer is usually already there.

Clinical Reflection

Search satisfaction ends inquiry at the moment of discovery, and what makes it treacherous is that the finding which stops the search is usually genuine. But a finding that is real and a finding that is sufficient are not the same. When a patient stays sicker than the answer accounts for, that gap is not noise. It is the diagnosis, still waiting. Ask when the finding first appeared, and whether the explanation fits the timeline — and, because some diagnoses live only in a history the patient is holding back, ask without judgment, in a room quiet enough that the answer has somewhere safe to land.

PART I — CHAPTER 5

Framing Effect

The Story You Inherit

The patient arrives with the frame already set. The frame tells you what to see. And — more quietly — what to stop looking for.

The consult note was three words. Failure to thrive. No mechanism. No timeline. No specific complaint. Just three words that managed to say everything and nothing simultaneously. Elias read them at the nursing station before he had seen her face.

She was eighty-one years old. Small. Neat, though less carefully than she once would have been. Her daughter stood near the window, arms crossed.

"She's just not herself," the daughter said. "She's stopped eating. She barely moves. She doesn't talk the way she used to."

Elias nodded. He was already inside the frame.

On rounds he looked at his notes before presenting. He had read the consult note three times. Failure to thrive. Something moved in him briefly — a habit forming its first question. What would make this not failure to thrive. He felt it start. Then the frame absorbed it. Three words that explained everything before anything had been examined had a particular gravity.

He presented what the label gave him. "Eighty-one-year-old female with progressive functional decline. Poor oral intake. Decreased mobility. Failure to thrive." The words came easily. Too easily. The frame held everything together, neatly, without friction.

At the bedside, Lighthouse did something Elias had not done. He pulled up a chair. Not the rolling stool that kept clinicians at a slight and useful distance. A chair. He sat at her level. He did not open the chart. He did not look at the monitor. He turned to her. He said nothing.

Then he asked one question.

"What hurts," he said.

The room changed. The woman looked at him with the expression of someone who has been waiting to be asked that very question.

"My back," she said. Her voice was thin but clear.

"And when did it start hurting," Lighthouse said.

She thought. "After I fell," she said.

The daughter turned from the window. "You fell."

The woman nodded slowly. "In the kitchen. A few weeks ago. I didn't want to worry anyone." Her hands moved slightly against the blanket. "I wasn't using my walker. You always remind me to use it even just to the kitchen. I didn't want you to know I hadn't. I didn't want to disappoint you."

The daughter's face changed. Not anger. Something closer to grief at having been, without meaning to, the reason her mother had decided silence was safer than honesty.

"Mom," she said softly. "You could never disappoint me."

The old woman studied her hands. "I'm sorry," she said.

Elias felt the frame cracking. Not dramatically. Not all at once. The way ice cracks before it gives way.

Back in the hallway, Lighthouse stopped.

"What did the admission note say," he asked.

"Failure to thrive," Elias said.

"And what did that tell you to look for," Lighthouse asked.

"Malnutrition. Depression. Cognitive decline. Social isolation."

"And what did it tell you not to look for."

Elias was quiet. He had known to ask the question. He had felt it form before the presentation even began. The label had been stronger. That was the thing he would sit with later — not that he had forgotten the question, but that he had felt it forming and then set it aside.

"Pain," Lighthouse said. "Failure to thrive is not a diagnosis. It is a description of someone who has stopped engaging with their life. Your job is to find out why."

The imaging was ordered that afternoon. A compression fracture. T12. Acute on chronic changes, consistent with a fall several weeks prior. Significant marrow edema. And on the chest film obtained alongside it, two healing rib fractures on the right side — eighth and ninth ribs, also consistent with the same fall. Three weeks of that pain had done the rest — the pounds lost, the muscle gone, the decline everyone had read as the diagnosis rather than its consequence. She had not stopped eating because she was failing. She had stopped eating because it hurt to sit up and hurt to take the breath that swallowing sometimes requires. She had not stopped moving because she was declining. She had stopped moving because movement was pain.

That evening Elias stopped by after the pain team had discussed options. She seemed lighter somehow. Not because the fracture had been fixed. Because someone had found it.

"I was embarrassed to admit it," she said. "The fall. I fall sometimes. I know I should use my walker." She looked at him. "I would have told someone sooner," she said. "If they'd asked."

Elias nodded. He did not say anything else.

Later that evening Lighthouse stopped in the doorway of the workroom.

"Failure to thrive," Lighthouse said. Elias looked up. "It is one of the most seductive phrases in medicine. Not because it is wrong." He paused. "Because it is comfortable. It gives everyone permission to stop asking questions and start managing decline." He watched Elias. "She did not have failure to thrive. She had a compression fracture, two broken ribs, and a daughter she loved too much to disappoint." He paused once more. "The frame was set before you entered the room. You carried it in with you. We all do."

He turned to leave. Then stopped.

"The antidote," he said, "is to ask the question that the label made unnecessary." He left.

That night Elias wrote in his notebook.

Failure to thrive is not a diagnosis.
It is a door closed before the search begins.
I knew the question.
I felt it forming. The label was louder.
Next time I will ask it anyway.

Clinical Reflection

Framing doesn't alter the facts; it alters which facts seem worth pursuing. An inherited label turns accurate observation into selective perception, and the most dangerous labels aren't diagnoses at all — whatever is actually wrong keeps generating the very picture the label describes, so each day it holds it looks more correct. The evidence against it is rarely hidden; it is filed under the frame. What breaks it is usually small: the one question the label made unnecessary, asked directly, at the patient's level, with the chart closed. Notice when the frame is doing the thinking. Then pull up a chair.

PART I — CHAPTER 6

Availability Bias

The Last Case

The mind reaches for what it remembers most easily.
Memory is persuasive.
The most dangerous diagnosis is the one
that looks exactly like the one you just saw.

The patient from yesterday was still with Elias. It had been the kind of case that stays with you. A young woman. Sudden collapse. Pulmonary embolism — a clot had broken loose and lodged in her lungs — caught at the last possible moment. The ICU team had nodded approvingly. The attending had said well done. Elias had replayed it twice before sleeping and once more on the walk in. He was still carrying it when he met the new patient.

Sixty-one years old. He had been carrying groceries up his own front steps when the breathlessness took him. His son drove him in, ran the last two red lights, and had not yet let go of his father's coat. Now he was sitting bolt upright on the gurney. Working to breathe. Sweat at his hairline despite the cool room.

"Started about an hour ago," he said, each word costing him something. "Out of nowhere. Can't catch my breath."

Sudden onset. No clear trigger. Tachycardic. Oxygen saturation eighty-eight percent on room air. The anxious stillness of someone whose body has told him something is terribly wrong.

It looked exactly like yesterday.

Pulmonary embolism rose in Elias's mind fully formed. Vivid. Insistent. The chest X-ray showed mild vascular congestion — nothing dramatic, nothing that argued strongly for one diagnosis over another. The EKG showed sinus tachycardia and nonspecific ST changes in the inferior leads. Easy to read as nothing at all to a resident already moving in a single direction.

On rounds, Elias presented with quiet urgency. "Sixty-one-year-old male with sudden onset dyspnea, hypoxia, and tachycardia. High concern for pulmonary embolism. CT angiogram ordered."

Lighthouse let the presentation land.

At the bedside, Lighthouse moved without hurry. The room was tense — a nurse drawing blood gases, oxygen being titrated upward, the controlled urgency of a team already certain of where this was going. Lighthouse listened to the lungs first. Crackles, bilateral, mid to upper lung fields. That alone did not rule out PE. But it did not particularly support it either.

He moved the stethoscope to the precordium. The room was loud. Monitors alarming intermittently. A respiratory therapist adjusting the oxygen mask. Lighthouse asked, without raising his voice of quiet. The room calmed slightly. He leaned closer.

Listened at the apex. Nothing loud. Something softer. Brief. Almost lost beneath the crackles and the monitor tones and the general motion of the room. He repositioned the patient slightly onto his left side. Listened again.

"There," he said.

He straightened. He did not say anything immediately.

In the hallway, he turned to Elias.

Elias had been so certain coming in that morning. He was still certain now. That was the thing he would not understand until later — that certainty and correctness are not the same.

"What did you hear at the apex," Lighthouse said.

Elias hesitated. He had listened — briefly, in the middle of titrating oxygen and reviewing the chest film and thinking about how quickly he could get the patient to the scanner. "I'm not sure I heard anything specific," he said.

"Go back," Lighthouse said. "Listen again, more carefully this time. Patient on his left side if he can tolerate it. But quickly."

He stood at the bedside a moment longer than necessary, thinking of a question he had heard asked in a different room two days ago.

What would make this not what I think it is.

He had not asked it this morning. The room had been too loud. So had his own mind.

"There's something there," he said slowly, returning to the hallway. "But it's quiet. I almost wouldn't have called it a murmur at all."

Lighthouse nodded. "In acute severe mitral regurgitation, the murmur is sometimes soft. Almost silent. This is not a failure of listening. It is physiology working against you."

He paused. "The most severe cases are sometimes the quietest. That is not intuitive. It is true."

The EKG was repeated. The inferior ST changes, dismissed thirty minutes earlier as nonspecific, now were more prominent. An inferior myocardial infarction. The posteromedial papillary muscle had infarcted along with the wall around it, and somewhere in the hour before he arrived, it had ruptured.

The echocardiogram confirmed it within minutes. Flail posterior mitral leaflet. Severe, acute mitral regurgitation. Pulmonary edema not from fluid overload but from a heart suddenly unable to move blood forward the way it had an hour before.

Cardiothoracic surgery and cardiology were called simultaneously.

Elias went back in. The monitor tones. The hiss of oxygen. The son standing with his back to the window. He addressed both of them.

"You have had a heart attack," Elias said. "A small one, on the back wall of the heart. But it damaged one of the muscles that holds a valve shut — the valve between the two chambers on the left side. This afternoon that muscle gave way. The valve is failing. Blood that should move forward is washing backward into your lungs. That is why you cannot breathe."

The son looked at his father. Then back at Elias.

"Can it be fixed."

"The surgeons can fix it. Tonight. The surgery has risk. But the bigger risk is in not fixing it."

The son nodded once, the way people nod when they have decided to believe you because the alternative is unbearable.

The patient was stabilized, an intra-aortic balloon pump placed and taken emergently to the operating room.

Elias stood outside the O.R. doors afterward, the way he was beginning to learn he often would in the aftermath of the cases that mattered most. Lighthouse found him there.

"It looked exactly like yesterday," Elias said.

"It was built to," Lighthouse said. "Acute MR from papillary rupture can present indistinguishably from PE in the first hour. Sudden dyspnea. Tachycardia. Hypoxia. A chest film that doesn't commit to one diagnosis over the other. The only difference was a murmur quiet enough to disappear into a room that was too loud and a mind that was already certain where it was going."

Elias thought of yesterday. The young woman. The collapse. The PE caught in time. "I wasn't wrong to think of PE," he said slowly.

"No," Lighthouse said. "PE belonged on the differential. It belonged at the top of it, given what he looked like in that first minute. The error wasn't including it. The error was stopping once you had a diagnosis that explained enough to stop you from listening carefully for the one finding that would have told you it was something else entirely."

That evening Lighthouse stopped in the doorway of the workroom. He turned to Elias. "The murmur was there from the moment he arrived. You didn't hear it because you were listening for confirmation of something you already believed, in a room that gave you every excuse not to listen carefully enough to hear it." He paused. "There is a question that would have slowed you down before the room got loud. You almost asked it today."

"What would make this not a PE," Elias said.

"Ask it before the room fills up," Lighthouse said. "Ask it before your mind does."

That night Elias wrote in his notebook.

What I remember most vividly is what I must listen past most carefully.
The room was too loud. So was I.
There is a question I did not ask.
Next time I will ask it first.

Clinical Reflection

Availability bias thrives on mimics. Some of medicine's most lethal conditions present, in their first minutes, as convincing copies of familiar ones — and the finding that separates them is sometimes the quietest thing in the room. Memory selects for drama, for the case that ended well because someone moved fast, but not every catastrophe announces itself the way the last one did. The correction is a quiet room and the willingness to ask — before the room fills and the mind follows — what would make this not the diagnosis I already believe it to be.

PART I — CHAPTER 7

Representative Bias

The Rash That Never Came

Diseases do not read textbooks.
They do not know how they are supposed to look.
The absence of a feature
is not the absence of a diagnosis.

Morning report began at seven-thirty. The room was full — coffee cups, overnight fatigue, and the alertness of people who had been through something and were not yet sure what it meant.

The presenting resident was thorough. He had been careful overnight, attentive, documented everything. He had not cut corners. He had simply looked for the wrong thing.

"Forty-four-year-old male," he began. "Transferred from a rural community hospital. Fever to one-oh-four. Severe headache. Diffuse myalgias. Confusion on arrival." He paused. "White count elevated. Platelets sixty-two thousand. Sodium one twenty-five. Liver enzymes elevated. No focal neurologic deficits. Chest X-ray clear. Blood cultures pending. LP unremarkable." He set down his paper. "We treated empirically for meningitis and possible viral encephalitis overnight. He remains critically ill."

Questions came from the room. Travel history. Exposures. Sick contacts. Medications. The resident answered carefully, completely, from his notes.

At the center of the room, Dr. Elara Holt listened without speaking. She was three years out from her own internship. Chief resident.

The kind of clinician who had learned that the most important thing you can do in a room full of tired people is listen for what isn't being said.

She looked at the numbers on the board. Platelets sixty-two. Sodium one twenty-five. Fever one-oh-four. She studied them together. Not separately. Something moved in her thinking.

In the back corner, Dr. Lighthouse sat in a chair he had taken when he arrived. He had not announced himself. He looked at the same numbers. "The sodium and the platelets," he said quietly — to no one, or perhaps to Elias, who sat nearby and heard him. Elias watched him. Lighthouse did not elaborate. Not yet.

Elara looked at the numbers one more time. Then she asked one question.

"What is the one diagnosis," she said, "that fits everything in this room. Not the fever alone. Not the platelets alone. Not the sodium alone. Everything. Together. All at once."

The room was quiet. Elias recognized the question. It had just arrived somewhere he had not yet reached.

"Tell me about the patient," Elara said.

The resident looked up. "I did," he said. Not defensively. Genuinely puzzled.

"Tell me about him. Not his labs. Him."

The resident thought. "He's an outdoorsman," he said slowly. "Hunting. Fishing. His wife said he's outside most weekends. Lives in a rural area."

Elara nodded. "And the rash," she said.

"No rash. We looked carefully. Multiple exams overnight. Nothing."

"Did you look between the fingers," she said. "Along the wrists. The ankles."

The resident hesitated. "I looked. There was nothing."

Elara had heard enough. She turned to the board and wrote two words beneath the lab values. Tick exposure. Then turned back to the room.

"Did anyone ask about tick exposure," she said.

A pause. "His wife said he hadn't mentioned any," the resident said.

"Hadn't mentioned," Elara said. She let that sit. "A man who hunts and fishes in rural countryside every weekend of his life does not report every tick to his wife. That is not the same as no exposure."

Elara turned back to the board. Beneath the three words she had written, she added one line.

Rocky Mountain Spotted Fever.

Then beneath it: No rash in up to fifteen percent of cases.

"The rash is the feature everyone waits for," she said. "It is also the feature that arrives last. Sometimes after the window for treatment has closed." She paused. "There was a paper in the *Archives of Internal Medicine*. Early nineteen eighties. They called it Rocky Mountain Spotless Fever. It was not a new disease. It was an old disease presenting without its most recognizable feature."

She set down the marker. "The textbook picture is not the only picture. It is simply the one we memorized."

The doxycycline was started within the hour, on clinical suspicion alone. By evening the fever had begun to break; by the next morning the man was asking for water, then food, then when he could go home. The PCR, when it returned, was positive for Rickettsia rickettsii — confirming what Elara had already treated.

After morning report had emptied Lighthouse remained in his chair at the back of the room. He had not spoken once during the discussion. Elara gathered her notes and felt him watching.

"Good work, connecting the low sodium and platelets," he said.

She looked up. "Together," she said. "In that patient. In that setting."

Lighthouse nodded slowly. "Each finding alone belongs to a lengthy list of diagnoses. Taken as one, in this patient, in this setting, the list becomes noticeably short." He paused. "That is always where to look. Not at what each finding means individually. At what they mean when you refuse to separate them."

He turned to her without a word. Then smiled. Not a large smile. Not effusive. The smile of a man who had spent a career waiting for people to see what he saw and had just watched someone do it without his help. Elara held it briefly. Then looked back at her notes.

That afternoon Elias found her writing in the workroom.

"How did you know where to look," he asked.

"The numbers didn't fit the diagnosis everyone was treating," she said. "Meningitis. Encephalitis. Neither one explains that platelet count and that sodium together. And he was an outdoorsman. Rural. Febrile. Critically ill without a clear source." She looked at Elias. "I asked myself what fits all of it. Not most of it. All of it."

"And the rash not being there," Elias said. "That didn't stop you."

"The rash not being there," Elara said carefully, "made me more suspicious. Not less. If the rash were there, someone would have found it overnight."

Elias stood in the doorway, thinking about a disease that had withheld its most recognizable feature and nearly gone unnamed because of it.

That night he wrote in his notebook.

The absent finding is not the absent diagnosis.
Ask what fits everything.
Not just what fits the picture.
That question travels further than I have gone yet.

Clinical Reflection

Representative bias mistakes the template for the truth. When a disease resembles a familiar pattern the mind stops questioning; when it doesn't, the mind stops looking. A single missing feature — the textbook finding everyone waits for — is often enough to remove a diagnosis from a room that has done everything else right. But the textbook picture is a composite, not a requirement, and diseases routinely withhold their most recognizable feature until the window to treat has closed. So don't discard the pieces when they fail to form the expected picture. Question the picture — and ask what single diagnosis fits everything in the room. Not most of it. All of it.

PART I — CHAPTER 8

Overconfidence Bias

The Confident Mind

Confidence is seductive.
Experience sharpens judgment.
It can also replace it.
The most vulnerable clinician
is the one who has stopped being surprised.

Elias had been right all week. That mattered more than he knew.

January had arrived the way it always arrived on the internal medicine service — without announcement and without mercy. Viral syndromes everywhere, wearing the same face, almost always leaving with the same diagnosis. Elias had moved through all of it with a fluency that surprised even him. Three correct diagnoses in a row, each story resolving cleanly in his hands before he had finished reading the chart. He had learned to trust that fluency.

The patient arrived just after noon. Fifty-five years old. A contractor. Arguing about the cost of an ambulance ride he wasn't sure he really had needed.

He was sitting on the gurney when Elias entered, hunched forward, one hand pressed to his temple. His color was off — a grayness beneath the skin that Elias noted without pausing on.

Headache. Nausea and vomiting. Fatigue. Cough. Dizziness. Confused this morning per triage note.

January. The flu everywhere. The story arrived fully formed before Elias had finished reading.

"When did this start," Elias asked.

"Two days ago," the man said. Then stopped to cough — dry, unproductive. "Maybe three. Hard to remember."

"Any fever,"

"Last night. I think."

"Anyone home with you sick too,"

"My wife's been at her mother's. Just me and the dog."

Temperature one hundred point six. Heart rate one-oh-eight. Blood pressure one-oh-two over sixty-eight. Oxygen saturation ninety-seven percent on room air — the reassuring number, the one that said not immediately dangerous and allowed the mind to move toward the more comfortable explanations.

Lungs clear. No focal findings. Neurological exam intact, though the man was slow to answer, his responses arriving a half-beat behind the questions. Elias attributed it to the headache and the fatigue and two days of vomiting.

The labs returned forty minutes later. Sodium mildly low. BUN elevated. Creatinine up from baseline. Mild metabolic alkalosis. Dehydration — clear and straightforward. The chemistry of a man who had been vomiting for two days and could not keep fluids down.

The picture was complete. Viral syndrome with significant dehydration. Admission for IV fluids, antiemetics, supportive care. A story that explained every finding on the page.

Elias wrote the admission note with the efficiency of a clinician who has seen this case before and knows where it ends.

He had moved the patient upstairs and was finishing the chart at the nursing station when the wife arrived.

She came off the elevator already talking, asking a passing nurse where her husband was, her voice carrying the urgency of someone who has spent the last hour in transit unable to do anything but worry. She had been flying back from her mother's. She had called the house from the airport when he didn't answer his phone, gotten no response, called a neighbor, and the neighbor had found him on the kitchen floor and called 911.

She found Elias at the station. "I'm his wife," she said. "What do you think is wrong."

"Most likely a viral illness," Elias said. "He is significantly dehydrated from the vomiting. We are admitting him for fluids and to get on top of the nausea."

She nodded, processing, still catching her breath. "Will he be all right,"

"We expect so," Elias said.

She looked toward the room, then back at him. "It's strange," she said. "The neighbor told me Daisy was right there next to him on the floor. Wouldn't get up. Hadn't touched her food." She shook her head slightly — the distracted shake of someone voicing a worry that feels small next to the larger one. "I don't know why I'm even thinking about the dog right now."

Elias had already started to close the chart.

He stopped.

Just me and the dog.

He thought of the question he had asked at triage — anyone home with you sick too — and the answer that had seemed, at the time, to close the question rather than open it. He thought of the dog now. Lethargic. Not eating. In the same house. Two members of the same household, sick in the same way, on the same timeline. One of them is a dog.

A viral syndrome did not explain the dog.

"Has the dog been sick recently," Elias asked. "Before today."

"No," the wife said. "She's never sick. That's why it's strange."

Elias stood very still. He thought of the chart he had just finished writing. Dehydration. Viral syndrome. A story that had explained every finding on the page and had, in doing so, explained nothing about the dog lying on the kitchen floor four miles away.

"I want to order a different test," he said, half to himself. He picked up the phone. "I need a co-oximetry panel. Not a standard sat. A co-oximetry. Now."

The result returned nineteen minutes later.

Carboxyhemoglobin twenty-four percent.

Elias studied the number. Then at the saturation reading still displayed on the monitor above the bed. Ninety-seven percent. He understood now what that number had been doing all along. The pulse oximeter had been accurate. It had simply been answering a different question than the one he thought he was asking.

He called the wife back to the desk. "I know what is wrong with him now. There is carbon monoxide in your house," he said. "Call your neighbor right now. Tell them to get the dog outside and call 911 from outside. Then don't go back in."

She was already reaching for her phone before he finished the sentence.

The fire department found a cracked heat exchanger in the furnace. Carbon monoxide had been leaking into the house for at least three days. The dog was taken to the emergency veterinary clinic by the neighbor — unsteady on her feet, head low, confused. She had been the first to know.

The husband was treated with high-flow oxygen and recovered without permanent neurological sequelae. The dog spent one night in an oxygen cage and was released by the following afternoon, eating again. The furnace was replaced before they could move back.

That evening Lighthouse found Elias in the workroom.

He sat down beside him. "The saturation was ninety-seven," Elias said. Not as an excuse. As an accounting.

"I know," Lighthouse said. "I read the chart." A pause. "What made you order the co-ox," he asked.

"The dog," Elias said. "Two members of the same household, sick the same way, on the same timeline. One of them a dog"

Lighthouse nodded. "A viral syndrome does not cross species," he said.

"No, it does not," Elias said.

"What made you stop and ask about it," Lighthouse said. "You had already finished. The chart was complete."

Elias considered this honestly. "It didn't fit," he said. "I noticed that it didn't fit, and I didn't have anywhere to put that yet, so I asked one more question instead of letting it go."

Lighthouse looked at him. "That is the whole of it," he said. "Not knowing the answer in advance. Noticing when something does not fit the answer you already have, and being willing to stop and ask one more question instead of filing it away."

He stood. "Confidence accumulates," he said. "It feels like clarity. After a week of viral syndromes, it feels like pattern recognition so reliable that the next case can be understood before it is fully heard." He paused at the door. "You had already closed the chart in your mind. The discipline was not in avoiding that. It is in staying willing to reopen it."

He left.

Elias sat for a long time. He thought of the dog on the kitchen floor, unable to tell anyone something was wrong, telling them anyway in the only language available to her. He thought of how close he had come to never hearing about her at all — if the wife had arrived ten minutes earlier or later, if she had mentioned it differently, if he had already moved on to the next patient. What could have happened if the three of them had moved back into that house unaware.

That night he wrote in his notebook.

The chart was already written.
But it did not explain the dog.
That is what stopped me —
not suspicion, but the discipline of noticing
what the answer I already had could not explain.

Clinical Reflection

Overconfidence does not announce itself. It accumulates in the space between a run of correct diagnoses and the next case — which deserves the same scrutiny and no longer seems to need it. A normal test reassures beyond its authority; the fact that would reopen the case often arrives sideways, in a remark from someone who doesn't know they are carrying it. The discipline is not avoiding closure — closure is how a service runs. It is noticing the one detail the answer cannot explain, and reopening a chart already written. The week you feel sharpest is the week to be most careful.

PART I — CHAPTER 9

Diagnosis Momentum

The Diagnosis That Traveled

Every handoff is a chance to reset.
Or a chance to stop thinking.
Momentum is not direction.
Certainty cannot be passed.
It can only be earned.

Morning report began at seven-thirty. The overnight resident presented with the exhaustion of someone who had been moving for twelve hours and was now being asked to be precise. He was precise. That was not the problem.

"Seventy-eight-year-old female," he began. "Brought in by ambulance from a rural satellite hospital last night. Working diagnosis sepsis of unclear source. Possible urinary. Fever to one-oh-three-point-eight. Altered mental status. Diffuse rigidity." He watched his notes. "White count elevated. Lactate mildly elevated. Blood cultures pending. Chest X-ray unremarkable. Urinalysis with mild pyuria." He paused. "Started on broad-spectrum antibiotics overnight."

He set down his paper.

Heads nodded. The story was familiar. An elderly woman. Fever. Confusion. Rigidity. A urinalysis with something in it. Sepsis. The diagnosis had traveled from the rural hospital note, to the E.R., to the admission note, and finally to the sign-out to this room. It was gathering confidence at every step the way diagnoses do when they go unquestioned across enough handoffs.

Dr. Elara Holt sat at the head of the table. Beside her, unexpectedly, sat Dr. Phillip Mann. Gastroenterologist. Senior attending. He had stopped by morning report on his way to an early endoscopy. He was a former chief resident of Dr. Lighthouse and had held morning report in this same room eight years before. He had no investment in the diagnosis already in motion. No note to defend, no decision to protect. He was simply a physician in a room full of physicians listening to a case with fresh ears.

At the back of the room, in a chair he had taken when he arrived late, sat Lighthouse. He had not announced himself. Elias sat nearby. He had watched Lighthouse arrive and say nothing and understood that this morning he was here to observe rather than to teach. That distinction, he was learning, was itself a form of teaching.

Elara looked at the overnight resident. "Tell me about her mental status on arrival," she said.

"Confused. Not following commands well. Daughter said she had been declining since yesterday morning."

"Any focal findings."

"No. Neuro exam limited by cooperation."

Elara was quiet. At the side of the table Dr. Mann leaned forward slightly. "The rigidity," he said. "Was it generalized or focal."

The overnight resident turned to his notes again. "Generalized," he said. "Though the nurse noted she seemed to have difficulty opening her mouth for the oral temperature."

"Difficulty opening her mouth," he said — not a question but a repetition that asked to be heard differently.

"It was documented as patient non-cooperation," the resident said.

Mann stood. He didn't speak at once. He walked to the whiteboard and looked at the word written at the top.

Sepsis.

He picked up the eraser. Held it. Then erased the word. Without explanation. Without theater.

At the back of the room, Elias went still. He had seen this before. The same room. A different word. A different hand holding the eraser. The same silence afterward.

Lighthouse watched from the back, silent.

Mann set down the eraser and turned to the room. "What has this diagnosis not yet asked," he said.

He studied Elara. She took it from there.

"It has asked about infection," she said. "It has asked about source. It has not asked about the patient's history before she arrived. It has not asked about wounds." She wrote three words on the board beneath the space where sepsis had been. Jaw. Rigidity. Fever. Then beneath them one more. Exposure.

She turned to the intern who had admitted the patient. "Call the daughter," she said. "Ask her one question. Has her mother had any cuts or wounds recently. Anything at all. No matter how small."

The intern left the room.

Mann spoke quietly into the silence. "When did you last see a case of tetanus," he asked the room. No one answered. "When did you last think about it," he said. Still no answer.

He was quiet. "I saw it more than once, a long time ago. Two years with the Peace Corps. West Africa. After my intern year. We did not practice medicine the way most of you know it now. Wound care wasn't always available. Vaccination coverage was inconsistent. I saw maybe a dozen cases in those two years. Farmers, mostly. A few children."

He paused. "You don't forget the jaw," he said. "Once you've seen it the first time, you don't mistake it for a patient who is simply uncooperative."

"Most of you have never seen it," he said. "That is not a failure of training. It is success. Vaccination programs have made it rare enough that most physicians practicing today will go an entire career without encountering it once." He looked around the table. "But rare is not the same as gone."

The intern returned four minutes later. She stood in the doorway. "The daughter says her mother cut her hand last week," she said. "Peeling a tomato. From her garden."

No one moved.

Elara looked at the whiteboard. Then added two words beneath what she had written. Garden soil. She turned.

"Clostridium tetani lives in the soil," she said. "It can survive on the surface of vegetables grown in contaminated ground. A minor wound is sufficient for inoculation. She is seventy-eight years old. She lives in the Amish community one county over, where tetanus vaccination is not routine. No documentation of immunization in her chart." She paused. "This is tetanus," she said.

Mann spoke once more. Quietly. Without theater. "The jaw tightness was trismus," he said. "It was in the notes." He paused. "Diagnosis momentum carried the sepsis label through every handoff with enough confidence that a cardinal feature of a different diagnosis was absorbed into it rather than stopping it."

He watched the overnight resident. Not unkindly. "The urinalysis gave everyone a place to stand. Mild pyuria in an elderly woman is common enough to be incidental. It became a source because the diagnosis needed one and it was available." He paused. "The momentum did the rest."

After the room emptied out, Lighthouse watched Mann set down the eraser. "I made you chief for a reason," he said. "You did," Mann said. "I'm still not sure you were right." "I was."

The team moved immediately. Tetanus immunoglobulin ordered. Metronidazole started. The patient was moved to a quiet room in ICU — tetanus patients are exquisitely sensitive to stimulation, sound and light triggering the spasms that are the disease's most threatening feature.

Elara went to see her before the transfer. She was a small woman. Neat even in illness. She kept a garden and used what it produced, and had never imagined that the soil she tended could carry something this old and this dangerous into her body through a knife cut on an ordinary afternoon. Her jaw was rigid. Her back arching slightly with each spasm.

Elara reached out and touched the woman's hand briefly. The woman could not turn her head. But her fingers moved. Just slightly.

After rounds Elara found Mann in the hallway outside the ICU. "The trismus was there on admission," she said.

"It was," he said.

"We almost missed it," she said.

"Yes," he said. "You almost did." He paused. "But you would have gotten there without me."

He looked at her. "The momentum stopped because someone in that room decided to ask what didn't fit instead of accepting what did."

She studied him. "You trained under Lighthouse," she said.

"A long time ago," he said.

"Did he teach you to look for tetanus," she asked.

Mann considered this. "He taught me to ask what the diagnosis in motion had not yet asked," he said. "I found tetanus on my own." He paused. "That is how it works. The question travels. What you find with it is yours."

Elias returned to the workroom. He turned to the whiteboard. Empty now. Clean. He thought of the board in the report room, and a word erased without explanation by a man in a pressed white coat on a July morning that felt like a long time ago. The same room where Mann had stood this morning. The same board. A different hand. A different word. He thought of Mann — a gastroenterologist who stopped by that morning, erasing a word he had never written.

The gesture had traveled from one room to another without anyone deciding to carry it. That was the thing about habits that were true. They moved on their own.

That night he wrote in his notebook.

Every handoff is a chance to reset.
The diagnosis you inherit is not the diagnosis you have earned.
Ask what the momentum has not yet asked.
The question travels. What you find with it is yours.

Clinical Reflection

Diagnosis momentum builds with every retelling. Each handoff adds confidence, each repetition removes doubt, and a diagnosis in motion does more than travel — it recruits: contradicting findings are absorbed rather than weighed, while the findings it needs are promoted past what the evidence justifies. The questions that halt it are the ones momentum never asks — about what came before arrival, about what the label has explained away rather than explained. And the person who asks them is usually the one with the least invested: no note to defend, nothing to lose by erasing a word someone else wrote. Inheriting a diagnosis is not the same as earning it.

PART I — CHAPTER 10

Time Pressure Bias

The Shortcut They Purchased

Urgency is not always the patient's.
Sometimes it belongs to the people who love them.
Or to the people who can afford to make it disappear.
The triage, the reassessment, the watching —
that is what cannot be bought back
once it has been traded away.

The emergency department was full. Not busy. Full. Every bay occupied. Hallway stretchers lined against the wall. The waiting room standing room only. The kind of night where triage becomes a form of triage itself — deciding not just who is sickest but who can wait the longest without becoming sicker while they do.

Elias came down to help with overflow. He saw them before he reached the desk.

A man in a tuxedo, black tie undone at the collar, the disarray of someone who had loosened it in irritation rather than comfort. A woman beside him in a long dark evening gown. Their son sat between them. College-age. Pale. Leaning back in the plastic chair rather than forward, shifting his weight every few minutes as though no position quite solved the problem, one hand resting low on his abdomen. Uncomfortable.

They had been pulled from an event. That much was obvious from fifteen feet away.

The father checked his watch. Not anxiously. Impatiently. "This is absurd," he said, not quite under his breath. "We are missing the entire dinner."

"Go, then," the mother said. "I want to stay with him." The tiredness of a woman who had already decided where she needed to be and had stopped negotiating about it. "I'll call you."

He stood. Straightened his jacket. "You're sure," he asked.

"Go," she said. "I promise I'll call."

He looked at his son — something between concern and irritation, neither one winning. Then he was gone, through the sliding doors, into a night he was already late for.

The mother sat beside her son, her hand on his back. She had chosen to stay when her husband chose to leave.

Elias almost approached them. Almost asked if they needed help. Before he could, his pager went off. Code blue. Seven east. He ran.

While he was gone, the father stopped in the parking structure on his way out and made a call. By the time Elias returned, twenty minutes later, it was already moving through channels he did not yet understand were moving above him.

The father did not call the triage desk. He called Doctor Turner, the hospital's Chief Medical Officer.

Elias learned about the call secondhand, the way residents learn about decisions made above them.

The attending found him at the workstation. "We're getting a direct admit," she said. "Eighteen-year-old male. Abdominal pain. He's being moved to the floor."

Elias looked up. He thought of the boy leaning back in his chair, his hand over his abdomen, the disease not yet declaring itself.

"He hasn't been triaged," he said.

"He's been evaluated," the attending said. "By his family's physician. Diagnosis is gastroenteritis. Fluids and observation overnight." She was already moving to the next task. "Get him settled. Start I.V. fluids for hydration. Labs in the morning." She paused. "The family has requested a Do Not Disturb order overnight. No vitals checks. No nursing checks between ten p.m. and six a.m. The father feels strongly that sleep is what the boy needs." She paused. "It's already been cleared. Turner called me himself."

She studied Elias. "Write the order," she said. It was not a request.

She left.

Elias examined the patient as best he could. Vague abdominal pain. Diffuse. Mild tenderness. No rebound he could elicit confidently. Low-grade fever. The story did not contradict gastroenteritis. It also did not confirm it.

"What did your doctor say exactly," Elias asked the mother.

"He said it was probably just a stomach bug. Something going around. He said fluids would do it."

"Did he examine him," Elias asked.

The mother paused. "He spoke to him on the phone," she said. "He's known him since he was born."

Elias wrote his note carefully. Diagnosis per family physician, phone consultation. Patient not examined by referring physician. Plan: intravenous fluids, overnight observation.

He read it back to himself. He thought about the triage process downstairs. The vital signs checked on arrival and repeatedly thereafter. The reassessment by different eyes at different hours. The nurse who would have noticed during the night if something had changed.

None of that was available now.

He ordered the labs for that evening. Not the morning. It was the only decision that remained entirely his. Then he wrote the order. No vital signs after nine p.m. No nursing checks between ten and six. He wrote it because he had been told to. He sat with it after he wrote it for longer than the task required.

The thing he had removed was not an inconvenience. It was the watching.

The labs resulted at eleven forty-seven. White count mildly elevated. Not dramatically. Not enough to act on urgently — not at midnight for a patient already labeled gastroenteritis, stable, observation, and not to be disturbed. Elias noted it. Filed it. Moved to the next patient.

The boy lay in a quiet private room where no one came to check whether the discomfort shifting in his abdomen was becoming something that needed to be seen before morning.

At six a.m. the order expired.

The night nurse went in. She came out quickly. He was worse. More focal now. The pain location was still vague. But he was less willing to move. Fever higher. Heart rate up. The vitals telling a story the evening vitals had been beginning to suggest and had been prevented from finishing.

Elias stood at the bedside and looked at the boy's face. Then at his abdomen. Then at the mother in the chair beside him, whose expression had shifted somewhere in the dark from worried to certain.

"He needs a CT," Elias said. He was already reaching for the phone. "I'm ordering it now."

The reply came back within minutes. The CT scanner on the floor had gone down overnight. A part failure. The only functioning scanner was in the emergency department, running its queue — trauma first, stroke alerts first, the acute and emergent ahead of the stable and admitted. A patient already on the floor, already labeled stable, already carrying a working diagnosis of gastroenteritis, joined that queue in the position his label earned him.

Which was not close to the front.

"When is the CT," the mother asked.

"They're working on it," Elias said.

He did not say that the patient had been displaced from the department where this scan would have happened hours ago. He did not say that the wait the family had spent considerable effort to avoid the night before was now being repaid with interest, at a moment when the disease had already used the intervening hours to advance unobserved.

The CT happened at twelve-fifteen.

Perforated appendix. Retrocecal. Periappendiceal abscess, established, not acute. The radiologist's note was precise: the degree of abscess organization suggested the perforation had not occurred during the hours of waiting on the floor. It had likely begun the previous evening. In a waiting room. Before any phone call had been made to anyone.

The disease had been progressing while the family negotiated his removal from the triage process that would have found it sooner.

Surgery was called. The operation was longer and more complex than it would have been with same-day imaging. The recovery would be too.

The father arrived just as his son was coming out of surgery. He walked through the doors and past the emergency department waiting room — the same plastic chairs, a different crowd — and down the corridor to the surgical waiting room. Quieter here. Carpeted. He sat beside his wife in his business suit this time. No tuxedo. No dinner.

The surgeon explained. The perforation. The abscess. The complexity of what had been a straightforward diagnosis the night before and was now a surgical recovery measured in weeks rather than days.

The father listened. Something had changed in him since the night before. He did not say anything. He sat with his wife and waited. This time without checking his watch — as if he had finally understood that there was nothing left to hurry.

Elias was in the workroom that evening when Lighthouse came in. He sat down without opening the chart.

"I was told to move him," Elias said. "Not asked. Told. The CMO had already called the attending by the time it reached me." He paused. "I ordered the evening labs myself. That was the only thing I did that wasn't already decided for me. Then I wrote the order. No vitals. No checks. The father felt strongly about it." He watched the table. "I wrote it because I was told to. And because I did not yet understand that what I was removing was not an inconvenience. It was the watching."

Lighthouse waited.

Elias looked up. "They thought they were buying him comfort," he said.

"They were buying him distance," Lighthouse said. "From the triage process. From the reassessment. From the nurse who would have come in during the night and noticed that something had changed. And the Do Not Disturb order completed what the private room began — it did not just move him away from the eyes that would have watched him. It instructed those eyes to stay closed."

Elias didn't answer.

"You could not have refused the admission," Lighthouse said. "The structure above you had already made that decision. That order was yours to write or not write."

Elias was very still. "I wrote it," he said.

"Yes," Lighthouse said. Not as condemnation. As the plainest possible acknowledgment of what had happened and what it meant.

After a while Lighthouse spoke again. "Remember tonight. Not because you could have stopped it. But because you will be the attending taking that phone call one day. When that day comes, remember what the triage process is actually doing before someone with the power to bypass it decides it is expendable."

He left.

That night Elias wrote in his notebook.

I wrote the order.
I could have refused it.
Bypassing the triage process avoid not just the waiting.
It avoids the watching.
I am writing this down, so I remember what it cost.

Clinical Reflection

Time pressure bias is usually pictured as a clinician moving too fast. Its quieter form is the opposite: a diagnostic process not rushed but bypassed — replaced, by someone with the standing to arrange it, with a conclusion optimized for comfort rather than certainty. The workup doesn't fail. It is never allowed to begin. What triage provides is not delay but surveillance — vital signs repeated, different eyes at different hours, a nurse who notices overnight that something has changed. A private room and a Do Not Disturb order cannot reproduce that vigilance; they can only remove it. The watching is the treatment.

PART I — CHAPTER 11

Outcome Bias

The Question That Felt Answered

A good outcome does not mean the reasoning was sound.
Sometimes the outcome is simply a question
that stopped being asked.
That is not the same as an answer.

He had been admitted for pneumonia. That was clear enough. Seventy-two years old. Productive cough. Fever to one-oh-three. Infiltrate on the chest film that left little room for argument. Antibiotics were started promptly. The kind of admission that proceeds the way admissions are supposed to.

By the second hospital day he was better. The fever came down. Not gone, but meaningfully lower — one-oh-one in the morning, one hundred by evening. He was eating a little. His color had improved. He was still confused, still slower than he should have been, but he was elderly and had been sick for several days, and confusion in an elderly hospitalized patient has a lengthy list of explanations that begins with exactly those two things. The chest film was improving at its edges. The antibiotics were working. The team relaxed.

When a treatment appears to be working, the question that produced it feels answered. That is the nature of outcome bias. Not laziness. Not carelessness. The reassurance of an intervention that does what it was designed to do, producing an improvement that confirms the thinking that preceded it.

The diagnosis had been correct. Everyone could feel it.

On the third hospital day a rash appeared on his scalp. Faint. Erythematous. Slightly raised in patches.

The resident examined it. "Drug reaction," she said. "He's on the new antibiotic. Common enough."

It was a reasonable conclusion. He was on a new medication. The rash had appeared after it was started. The antibiotic was switched. The rash was documented, explained, and filed under a question that now had an answer.

Why does he have a rash. Antibiotic allergy.

The question closed. It closed easily because the room was already in the posture of a team whose diagnosis had been confirmed by improvement. Nobody asked it again.

On the fourth hospital day he seized. Generalized. Brief. Resolved with lorazepam.

"Any history of alcohol use," the attending asked the family.

His daughter hesitated. "He has a drink most evenings. I don't know how much exactly."

That was enough. Alcohol withdrawal seizure. Common in a hospitalized elderly patient several days removed from his usual routine. The benzodiazepine had worked. The seizure had stopped.

Why did he seize. Withdrawal.

An Alcohol Withdrawal (CIWA) protocol was initiated. Scheduled benzodiazepines added. The question closed again. And again the closure came easily — because the room was managing complications in a patient who was otherwise improving. Nobody connected it to the rash. They were, after all, two separate questions. Each one already answered.

The pneumonia was getting better. That was the fact the room kept returning to.

On the fifth hospital day the fever climbed again. One-oh-two by evening. Then one-oh-three. This was attributed to the pneumonia — a common pattern, a dip followed by a secondary rise as the inflammatory cascade worked itself out. The antibiotics were broadened. He was more confused now than he had been on admission. More disoriented. Agitated, at times combative with the nurses — what the ward still called hospital psychosis, the familiar unraveling of an elderly man several days into an unfamiliar bed. This too was attributed: to the fever, to the disrupted sleep, to the accumulated effect of several days in a hospital bed — and to the benzodiazepines running on the withdrawal protocol, which could cloud an old man further even as they were meant to settle him.

The explanations were available. They were applied. They fit well enough that nobody felt the need to look further.

The pneumonia was still the diagnosis. The improvement of day two was still the proof.

Lighthouse saw him on the sixth day. A teaching attending, rounding with the team on a service he did not usually carry, covering for a colleague.

"We usually just do chart rounds on the older admissions," the resident said. "I don't," Lighthouse said. "I read the chart. Then I see the patient."

He read the chart carefully before entering. Pneumonia, improving on day two, then complicated. Rash attributed to drug reaction, antibiotic switched. Seizure attributed to alcohol withdrawal, CIWA protocol running. Fever returning, antibiotics broadened. Three findings — rash, seizure, returning fever — each one absorbed into the pneumonia story or filed under its own separate answer. None of them asked to account for the others. None of them allowed to raise a question the improvement of day two had already seemed to answer.

He went in.

He examined the patient. Still confused. More than the fever alone should explain. More than hospital delirium in an elderly man should look like by the sixth day. He looked at the rash. It had spread slightly since the antibiotic was switched. Still confined to the scalp and upper forehead. Still erythematous. But something else now. Vesicular. Small fluid-filled lesions among the erythema, easy to miss if you were looking for the resolution of a drug reaction rather than looking at what was there.

He paused. Then asked the resident one question.

"Is the rash unilateral or bilateral," he said.

The resident looked. Looked again, more carefully. "Unilateral," she said slowly. "Left side. I hadn't noticed that before."

"Drug reactions are typically symmetric," Lighthouse said — an observation, not a correction, the kind that invites a different question rather than closing the one already asked.

He turned to the patient. Confused. Febrile despite broadened antibiotics. A unilateral vesicular rash that had not resolved when the offending antibiotic was stopped. A seizure on hospital day four — later than classic withdrawal timing. A fever that had climbed rather than fallen as the pneumonia appeared to improve.

Three findings. Each given its own satisfying answer. The improvement on day two had made all of those answers feel secure. None of them had been asked to explain the others.

"I think this is herpes zoster," Lighthouse said. "Affecting the trigeminal distribution." He paused. "And I am concerned it has gone further than the skin."

No one spoke.

"Encephalitis," he said.

The lumbar puncture was performed within the hour. Elevated white count in the cerebrospinal fluid. Lymphocytic predominance. PCR sent for varicella zoster virus. It returned positive the next day.

Herpes zoster encephalitis.

Acyclovir was started empirically the moment the LP results suggested a viral process. The delay from rash to recognition had been three days — three days during which a treatable encephalitis had been masked not by the pneumonia alone, but by the early improvement that had made the pneumonia feel confirmed, and by two subsequent findings that had each been given their own explanation rather than being asked what they shared.

He survived. The hospitalization extended significantly. A rehabilitation stay followed. He went home. Slower than he had been. Different than he had been. But home.

That evening Lighthouse stood with the resident in the workroom. She had been quiet since the LP results returned.

"The antibiotics worked," she said. "He got better on day two. That felt like proof."

"It was proof," Lighthouse said. "Of the pneumonia. He had pneumonia. The antibiotics treated it." He paused. "That is what outcome bias does at its quietest. It does not require a wrong diagnosis. It requires only a correct one, followed by an improvement, followed by a room that has stopped asking questions because the improvement answered them."

He sat down across from her. "The rash came after the improvement. The seizure came after the improvement. The returning fever came after the improvement. Each one arrived into a room that had already been reassured. Each one was given the most available explanation and set aside. Nobody asked what they had in common. Nobody asked that question because the improvement had already answered the larger one."

"How did you know to ask it," she said.

"I didn't carry the improvement with me," Lighthouse said. "I read the chart fresh. I saw three findings without their explanations attached. They looked different that way." He paused. "Sometimes that is all it takes. Not more knowledge. Less investment in the answer the outcome already provided."

The resident did not write a clinical pearl that night. She wrote one question and let it stand alone.

When the outcome reassures the room,
ask what the room has stopped looking for.

She did not show it to anyone. Some lessons are written for an audience of one.

Clinical Reflection

Outcome bias needs no wrong diagnosis — only a correct one, followed by an improvement, followed by a room that has stopped asking questions because the improvement answered them. And improvement does something quieter still: it lowers the standard of proof for everything after, so new findings are dispositioned rather than investigated. When a patient produces more than one new finding after an initial improvement, resist the pull of the improvement.

Ask what the new findings have in common — what single process could account for all of them at once. The improvement told you the first diagnosis was right. It did not tell you the story was finished.

PART I — CHAPTER 12

Hindsight Bias

The Obvious Answer

After the fact, everything makes sense.
That does not mean it was obvious.
It only means the story
has finally finished being told.

She had been seen five times in two weeks. That was the fact nobody could ignore once the diagnosis was known. Five times. Two emergency department visits, an oncology follow-up, and an ENT consultation. Then back to the ER a third time. Five sets of notes. Five clinicians who had listened carefully, examined thoroughly, and sent her home with an explanation that did not match what her body was doing.

In retrospect it would seem impossible. In retrospect it always does.

She was seventy-two years old. Simply dressed — a cotton sundress, the kind she apparently wore in every season, a small woman whose economy of presentation had nothing to do with indifference and everything to do with a life organized around what mattered. She walked with a cane, the unhurried gait of someone who had been managing a body that required accommodation since childhood. Polio, her chart noted briefly, age four.

The first emergency department visit had been for sinus fullness. Mild facial pressure. Three to four weeks duration. Antibiotics prescribed. Fluids recommended. Reassurance given. The second visit three days later — worse, not better. Sinus X-ray normal. Antibiotics changed. Follow-up advised.

Then her oncology appointment — routine, coincidentally timed. A history of endometrial carcinoma, treated five years prior, presumed cured. The port-a-cath was there, visible just below her clavicle — a small reservoir under the skin, its slender catheter resting in the great vein that carries blood from the head and arms back to the heart. Placed for chemotherapy. Left in when treatment ended.

It was documented in the note. It was not examined. It was not connected to anything. She told her oncologist her symptoms. He nodded as if he understood.

Her oncologist referred her to ENT the same afternoon. Exam normal. Nasal steroid inhaler prescribed.

Two days later she returned to the emergency department. The fullness in her face had become pressure. The pressure had spread into her neck. She was sleeping propped up now because lying flat made everything worse — but no one had thought to ask her that question.

The nurse practitioner who saw her that afternoon was exasperated. She was busy. The department was full. The chart showed three prior encounters for the same complaint with three reasonable explanations already applied. She told her to go home and take her medications. She said, more sharply than she perhaps intended, that the emergency department was not the place for chronic sinus problems.

The woman thanked her quietly. Without protest. She left.

She sat in her car in the parking structure for a few minutes, her cane across her lap. She knew where she needed to go. She had known, if she was honest with herself, since the second visit. That someone along the way would find it. That she would not have to be the patient who showed up at a doctor's office without an appointment, tearful, asking for help that the system had already declined to give her five times.

But she knew Lighthouse. Not well. From her cancer treatment, five years ago. She had seen him that once in consultation. She could not remember why. But she knew his reputation. Enough to know that if anyone would listen — really listen, the way she had watched him listen to her and to other patients in the clinic — it was him.

She drove to the building where she knew he had his office. She asked the woman at the desk if she could please speak with Dr. Lighthouse. She was crying when she said it. Not about the sinus pressure or the two weeks of visits. She was crying because nobody had believed her and she was tired and frightened and she had saved the one thing she trusted most for last.

Lighthouse was with a patient. He asked Elias to see her first.

She sat down carefully in the chair across from the desk — not on an examination table, in the chair, in his office, the choice of a woman who had not come for an examination and was not sure she was entitled to one. Her cane rested against the armrest beside her. She was flushed. Not the flush of embarrassment, though she was embarrassed. Something more fixed than that. A redness in her face that had settled in rather than risen.

She told the story. The sinus fullness. The five visits. The medications that had not helped. The nurse practitioner that afternoon.

"She told me to stop coming in," she said. She paused. "Nobody believes an old woman." She said it without self-pity. As a fact she had arrived at over the preceding two weeks through a process of elimination.

Elias listened. He looked at her face. The flush was fixed, bilateral — not the kind that came and went. He studied her neck. Something there, subtle, that he noted without yet naming. He reviewed the chart quickly. The port-a-cath was documented across every note. Present each time. Unremarked upon each time.

He asked about the sinus fullness. About the antibiotics. About the ENT visit.

He did not ask what made it worse.

He was not yet sure what he was looking at. He went to find Lighthouse.

They went back in together.

Lighthouse looked at her the way he watched patients — not at the chart, not at the monitor. At her. Then at her face. Then at her neck. He leaned forward slightly, and Elias looked again at what he had seen and half-registered and not yet named.

The veins. Subtle. The distension of vessels that have nowhere to drain.

Lighthouse looked just below her clavicle. The port-a-cath was there — a small elevation beneath the skin, visible above the neckline of her sundress. Five years old. Placed for chemotherapy. Left in when treatment ended.

"What makes it worse," Lighthouse said.

She looked slightly surprised. Nobody had asked her that. "Lying down," she said. "It's much worse when I lie flat. I've been sleeping in the chair for three days."

Elias felt the diagnosis arrive. Not gradually. All at once. The flush. The neck veins. The port. The positional worsening. A woman whose face felt full and whose symptoms climbed when she was supine and who had a foreign body sitting in the path of her superior vena cava — that same great vein — that nobody had thought about because everyone was focusing on her sinuses.

"The port," he said. Quietly. Almost to himself. Lighthouse looked at him. Nodded. Waited. "Superior vena cava obstruction," Elias said. "The port is the source. A thrombus. The positional worsening, the facial flushing, the neck veins —" He stopped. "It's all one thing," he said.

Lighthouse had what he needed. He turned back to her — the directness of a man who has just confirmed what he already believed and is now doing the thing that medicine sometimes asks of you, not the diagnosis, not the treatment, but the moment before both of those, when a patient who has not been believed for two weeks needs to hear something true from someone she trusts.

"Your port has developed a small clot on it. Enough to obstruct the vein draining blood from your head and arms. Your head is like a giant balloon steadily filling up. We are going to solve this today," he said. He paused. "And you will be better by tonight."

She began to cry softly. "That is exactly how it feels. Like my head just keeps building up pressure. I know now why I had to get to you. I know I can trust you," she said — not gratitude so much as the plain statement of a fact she had been holding onto since she sat in her car in the parking structure with her cane across her lap.

Lighthouse called the chief of oncology directly. He explained the case without preamble. The port. The two weeks of symptoms. The multiple visits. ER twice, Oncology, ENT then back to the ER today. The positional worsening. The facial flushing. The neck veins.

On the other end of the line a brief silence. "Who is her oncologist," the chief said, with a slight disdain. Not of Lighthouse, but of whoever could have missed something so obvious.

"One of your junior partners," Lighthouse said.

Another silence. Shorter than the first. Then he said sharply, "Send her to see me. Only me. Now."

The imaging confirmed it within the hour. A thrombus, extensive, compressing the superior vena cava at the site of the port-a-cath. The carcinoma had not recurred. The hardware placed to treat it had, in its own quiet way, nearly finished what the disease had not.

The thrombectomy was performed by interventional radiology that afternoon. She was better by evening. And the symptoms mostly resolved by the next day.

That evening Elias pulled up the five prior notes. Read them in sequence.

The port-a-cath was documented in every single one. Present. Unremarked upon. A detail that had traveled through Five clinical encounters without once being connected to the symptom sitting directly above it. The positional worsening was not in any of them. Nobody had asked.

He thought of his own examination that afternoon. He had seen the flush. He had noticed the neck veins without quite naming them. He had reviewed the chart. He had not asked what made it worse. He had gone to get Lighthouse instead — which was the right call, and the thing that stayed with him, the discomfort of recognizing how close he had come and where he had stopped.

He thought of the woman in the chair with her cane beside her. He thought of what she had said. Nobody believes an old woman. He thought of what it meant that she had saved Lighthouse for last.

Lighthouse stopped in the doorway.

"The port was in every note," Elias said.

"Yes," Lighthouse said.

"And the positional worsening. Nobody asked."

"No," Lighthouse said. He came in. Sat down. "Now that you know the diagnosis," he said, "how does it look."

Elias thought about this honestly. "Obvious," he said.

"Yes. It does now." He paused. "Was it obvious."

"No," Elias said. "Not without asking about position. Not without looking at the port as a potential source rather than a historical detail."

"Then do not pretend it was," Lighthouse said. "Hindsight bias does not only distort how we judge the past. It distorts how we learn from it. If we tell ourselves the diagnosis was obvious, we learn the wrong lesson. We do not learn to ask the question that would have made it one."

He turned to Elias. "What is the question," he said.

"What makes it worse," Elias said.

Lighthouse nodded. "Four words. Not in any of the five notes. Not because anyone forgot to ask. Because the sinus explanation had already decided the diagnosis." He stood. "She had been sleeping in a chair for three days. Nobody asked her why."

He paused. "She saved me for last," he said. Without pride. With the weight of a man who understands what it means to be someone's last option and what that asks of you when they finally arrive. "That is not a compliment," he said. "It is a responsibility." He left.

That night Elias wrote in his notebook.

Someday someone will save me for last.
I want to know what that asks of me before they arrive.

Clinical Reflection

Hindsight bias distorts not only how we judge the past but how we learn from it. Once a diagnosis is known the path to it looks straight, and the clinicians who missed it look careless. They were not. They applied the most available explanation to the findings they had. The clue is rarely hidden; more often it is documented, copied faithfully forward, and never once examined — a finding transcribed at every encounter has not necessarily been thought about at any of them. Judge every decision by the information available when it was made. Then find the question that was missing, and make it yours.

Part II

When Thinking Fails

By the time clinicians become skilled, their mistakes change. They no longer miss diagnoses because they do not know enough. They miss them because they know too much. Patterns form quickly. Stories resolve early. Explanations arrive before the patient finishes speaking.

This part of the book is about that moment — the moment when thinking becomes smooth, when coherence feels comforting, when uncertainty feels unnecessary. The cases here are not harder because the diseases are rarer. They are harder because they are messier. They resist clean explanations. They contradict themselves. They refuse to behave. And the errors they contain no longer belong to individuals alone. They belong to teams, to rooms, to protocols, to the accumulated weight of agreement — failures that feel, while they are happening, exactly like good medicine.

Elias Ward is a resident now, learning that teaching is harder than knowing. Maya Chen is the new intern, watching him the way he once watched someone else. The question that carried Part I — what does not belong — is still necessary. It is no longer sufficient. The question this part asks is quieter and harder.

What are you trying to make fit.

PART II — CHAPTER 1

Narrative Coherence Bias

The Story That Fit Too Well

A good story
Is not the same as a true one. When the pieces fit too well,
Something may have been erased.
Sometimes that something is the truth

Elias had been a resident for exactly seven days when Maya Chen started her first ER rotation. She had begun internship a week late — married in late June, just before the year started, and still away when the others began. She was sharp, quiet in the way of someone still deciding when it was safe to speak. She had been assigned to him for the next two months.

He had not yet decided what kind of teacher he wanted to be. He would learn something about that tonight — not by choosing it, but by failing at it first. Elias did not know yet that he would remember this shift for the rest of his career.

The patient was forty-eight years old. Chest discomfort. Burning, he said. Worse after eating. Worse lying down. He had a history of reflux. Took an over-the-counter antacid most days. Had run out two weeks ago and never refilled it.

Elias listened to the account. It fit. Burning quality. Postprandial worsening. Positional component. A known history. A lapsed treatment. The EKG was unremarkable. Troponin negative. Blood pressure one forty-two over eighty-eight. Elevated. Consistent with pain and anxiety.

He did not check the other arm. The story had not asked him to.

Maya stood beside him at the chart. "What do you think," she asked.

"Acid reflux, GERD," Elias said. He said it cleanly — the diagnosis arrived without friction, explaining everything the patient had described. He reached for the question he had been carrying since July. What would make this not GERD. He held it. The account looked back at him without flinching. Postprandial burning. Positional worsening. Known history. Lapsed treatment. The question found nothing that did not fit.

That should have been the warning. A case that answers every question you know to ask is not complete. It has only learned to wear the shape of completion. He did not understand that yet.

"Give him something for the reflux," Elias said. "Discharge with instructions to follow up with his primary care doctor if it doesn't improve."

Maya wrote the prescription. Something about the visit sat with her in a way she could not name. Not a clinical instinct. Something quieter — the sense that a story had resolved itself a little too easily. She did not say anything. She did not yet trust the things she could not name. She would learn to.

The patient thanked them on his way out. The explanation felt finished. That was the problem.

Twenty-four hours later he came back by ambulance.

Elias was back on shift. He did not recognize the name immediately. Then he did. The same man. Different now. Pale. Diaphoretic. Pain radiating to his back in a way it had not twenty-four hours earlier. Blood pressure asymmetric between his arms — a finding nobody had checked on the first visit because the case had not asked for it and because the explanation had already felt complete.

Elias felt the floor shift slightly beneath the case.

"Tell me what's different," he said. His voice steadier than he felt.

"It's not the same pain," the man said, breathing carefully. "This is tearing. Through to my back."

Maya stood beside him again. She had been on shift too. Had seen the chart from the night before. Recognized the name at the same moment Elias had. She did not say anything. She watched him.

The CT angiogram was ordered within minutes. The images came back at eleven-forty. Type A aortic dissection, extending from the aortic root into the descending aorta. Cardiothoracic surgery was called emergently. The patient was taken to the operating room within the hour.

Elias sat at the workstation afterward. He pulled up his own note from the night before and read it slowly.

Burning quality. Postprandial worsening. Positional component. History of GERD. EKG unremarkable. Troponin negative. Likely reflux exacerbation.

Every word of it had been true. He had not invented anything. He had simply stopped once the account closed itself. He had not asked what a dissection might feel like in its earliest hours, before it tears far enough to announce itself with radiation to the back. He had not checked blood pressures in both arms. He had not asked whether this pain felt different from any reflux the patient had experienced before.

The account had been coherent. Coherence had been the trap.

Maya found him there. She sat down across from him the way Lighthouse sometimes sat across from Elias, though she did not yet know that gesture had a history.

"The story fit," she said quietly. Not as accusation. As something closer to disbelief — the specific disbelief of watching your first teacher turn out to be capable of the same error you had been taught to fear in yourself.

"It did," Elias said. "It wasn't a bad diagnosis. It was an incomplete one that felt complete because it didn't leave anything unexplained." He looked at her. "That's different from being right," he said.

Lighthouse found them an hour later. He sat down — a third person at a small table that had become, without anyone deciding it, a place where difficult things were allowed to be said slowly.

"Walk me through it," he said to Elias.

Elias did. The burning pain. The postprandial pattern. The history. The clean diagnosis. The return twenty-four hours later. The asymmetric pressures nobody had thought to check the first time.

Lighthouse listened without interrupting. "A coherent account," he said, "is not evidence of a correct diagnosis. It is evidence that you stopped asking what didn't fit once you found something that did." He studied Elias. "Early dissection borrows the language of more common things before it commits to its own. What you were told was not a lie. It was incomplete, and completeness is not something a patient can offer you. It is something you have to look for, even when the story has already answered every question you thought to ask."

Maya had been listening carefully. Her first rotation as an intern. Watching her first teacher walk through the humility of his first real error — not as an abstraction but as a man now in an operating room fighting for his life.

"How do you know when a story is too clean," she asked.

Lighthouse considered the question. "You don't, not reliably," he said. "That is why the discipline isn't suspicion. It's the habit of asking one question the explanation doesn't need in order to make sense. A blood pressure in the other arm. Whether this pain resembles anything the patient has felt before. Something that costs almost nothing and changes everything when the answer is the one you were not expecting." He stood. "The story will always feel complete. That is what stories do. Your job is to ask one more question than the story requires."

He left them at the table.

That night Elias opened his notebook.

The account was true.
Every part of it. It was also incomplete.
Ask one more question than the story requires.
That is the only promise that has ever actually held.

Clinical Reflection

Narrative coherence bias is not a failure to gather information. It is the failure to see that a complete-feeling story is not the same as a complete one. Everything the patient reports can be genuine and still fit something else entirely, because dangerous conditions in their earliest hours often borrow the language of common ones before committing to their own. A story should not be trusted because it explains everything. It should be tested by one question it was never asked to answer — a pressure in the other arm, whether this pain resembles anything the patient has felt before — something that costs almost nothing and changes everything when the answer is the one you weren't expecting.

PART II — CHAPTER 2

Narrative Compression

The Interrupted Story

When you summarize too early,
you decide what matters.
Everything else disappears.
The patient already knows this.
That is often why they keep talking.

The patient spoke slowly. The type of slowness that makes a busy resident try to finish every sentence for the patient.

He was sixty-eight years old. Diarrhea, persistent. Fatigue. Weight loss. His account wandered. Symptoms overlapped. Timelines blurred. Details contradicted each other in the way real memory does when it has not been asked to perform for anyone before.

Elias felt the familiar urge. To organize. To clarify. To help.

"So, the diarrhea started after the antibiotics," Elias said.

The patient hesitated. "Well — maybe before," he said. "It's hard to remember exactly. There was a lot going on in my life then. My wife was ill."

Elias nodded. He wrote it down anyway, in the cleaner version that had already formed in his mind somewhere between the question and the answer he had wanted.

Maya stood at the foot of the bed. She had been with Elias for three weeks now — long enough to recognize his rhythms, the way he listened, attentive but already moving toward the shape he expected the account to take. She had watched him be wrong once already, on her first night, in a way that had changed how carefully she watched him since. She listened now for the thing that didn't quite fit.

On rounds, Elias presented efficiently. "Sixty-eight-year-old male with persistent diarrhea and weight loss. Symptoms began following a course of antibiotics for a prior sinus infection. Outside CT was normal two weeks ago. The screening test for Clostridium difficile was positive. Concern for antibiotic-related colitis."

The presentation sounded clean. The attending nodded. The plan moved forward.

Maya did not say anything in the moment. She was still learning when silence was patience and when it was complicity.

At the bedside afterward, the patient frowned slightly. "That's not exactly what I meant," he said.

Elias smiled, reassuring. "It's okay," he said. "I understand."

He did not ask him to continue.

Maya watched the patient's face in the half second after Elias spoke. Something passed over it. Not relief. The flatness of someone who has tried twice to say something and has twice been gently redirected toward a version of himself that was easier to chart.

In the hallway, Maya caught up to Elias. "I thought he said the diarrhea started before the antibiotics," she said. She kept her voice even.

Elias paused. "That's not how it came across," he said.

"Maybe," Maya said. "But he kept trying to explain it. Twice."

Elias considered this. He thought of his own chart, eleven days into residency, a man with chest pain that had also seemed to explain itself cleanly enough to stop him from asking one more question.

"What do you think we're missing," he said. It was not quite an apology. It was closer to a door, left open rather than closed. Maya did not yet have an answer. But she noticed that he had asked.

The workup proceeded along the path the compressed history had set for it. The C. diff screen had come back positive that morning — confirming what everyone already believed. Not just a coherent account now but one with laboratory support.

Treatment was started. The outside CT was not repeated.

Then the confirmatory PCR test for C. diff came back negative. A more sensitive test contradicting the initial result. The team paused. Briefly. The diarrhea could still be antibiotic-related without true C. diff infection. The positive screen could be a false positive. Maybe the PCR was a false negative. The timeline still fit. The diagnosis drifted forward anyway, carried less by evidence now than by the momentum of having already been written into enough notes that questioning it felt like more work than the negative result seemed to demand.

Maya returned to the room alone that evening, between other tasks. She sat down. She did not open her notes. She looked at him.

He looked back — the look of a patient deciding whether this visit was going to be like the others or whether something had changed.

"Can you tell me again," she said, "about when the diarrhea started."

He watched her carefully. "You actually want to know," he said. It was not quite a question.

"I do," Maya said. She sat back slightly. She did not write anything yet.

He talked for nearly twenty minutes.

The diarrhea, he said, had started before the antibiotics. Months before. Loose stools, intermittent at first, then more frequent, accompanied by cramping and a gradual loss of appetite he had attributed to stress. The antibiotics had come later, for an unrelated sinus infection, and the timing had simply overlapped — so when the diarrhea worsened, he had assumed, as the doctors seemed to assume, that the antibiotic was the cause. But the diarrhea had been there first.

"Nobody really wants the long version," he said. "They want the part that explains it quickly."

Maya brought it to Elias the next morning, offering it as information, not correction.

"I went back and asked him to tell me everything," she said. "Not just the part about the antibiotics." She showed him her notes.

Elias read them slowly. The four-month history. The early appetite loss. The diarrhea that predated the event everyone had organized the entire workup around. The colonoscopy never done.

"That changes things," he said.

A CT was ordered that afternoon — this time with the actual timeline in mind. The outside study, done two weeks earlier, had been negative. This one was not. A mass in the ascending colon. Four months of intermittent diarrhea and progressive weight loss, explained at last by something that had never had anything to do with antibiotics.

Colon cancer. Locally advanced but not yet metastatic. Resectable.

That evening Elias found Maya in the workroom. He sat down across from her.

"You went back," he said.

"I did," Maya said.

"Why."

She considered the question. "Because he tried to tell us twice," she said, "and we both decided the shorter version was easier to work with."

"I did that," Elias said. "Not you."

"I didn't stop you," Maya said.

"You came back," he said. "That's different." He paused. "I keep thinking about my first week. The man with the chest pain. Everything he told me was true. I just stopped asking once it added up to something I recognized." He looked at her. "You asked one more question than the story required. That's the only thing that ever actually works."

Maya thought about this. "It wasn't really one question," she said. "It was the same question, twice. The second time, I just stayed long enough to hear the answer."

That night Elias wrote in his notebook.

Compression is not a failure of listening.
It is a failure of staying.
The story the patient offers first
is the one they believe you can hear.
Stay until they believe you can hear the rest.

Clinical Reflection

Narrative compression begins not with bad intentions but with the wish to organize a patient's account into something a busy team can act on. The patient offering a more complicated, more accurate version twice is not being evasive — he is being edited. A confirming lab completes the trap: a positive test inside an already coherent story ends scrutiny rather than inviting it. By the time a better test contradicts the first, the story has been written into enough notes that questioning it feels like more work than the result seems to demand. The antidote is to return, when something doesn't sit right, and ask the same question a second time — then stay long enough to hear the answer that doesn't come in the first thirty seconds.

PART II — CHAPTER 3

Cognitive Dissonance

The Patient Who Would Not Make Sense

The pause is not empty.
It is where the second answer arrives.
The first answer is often the one the room is ready to hear.
The truth may need someone to stay.

The labs did not agree. Sometimes they do not. The key is what you do when they refuse to cooperate.

The patient was sixty-one years old. Recurrent fevers. Weight loss. Diffuse pain that moved from one place to another without any pattern Elias could find. Blood cultures, negative. Imaging, unrevealing. Autoimmune serologies, inconsistent — one mildly positive, repeated and negative the next time, as though the body itself could not decide what story it wanted to tell. Nothing resolved.

Elias reviewed the chart again. And again. Each time the same low current of irritation rose in him. The data should have converged by now. It did not.

On rounds he presented carefully. "Sixty-one-year-old male with prolonged febrile illness. Extensive workup, largely unrevealing. Symptoms remain difficult to characterize." The words felt thin. Unsatisfying in the way that an honest presentation of an unsolved case always is.

At the bedside, the patient spoke haltingly. "Some days it's my joints," he said. "Other days it's my stomach. Then it's gone for a while. I know that doesn't make sense."

Elias nodded. He felt the tension rise in his own chest before he had decided to let it. "That's not typical," he said.

The patient looked down. "I know," he said. "I wish it made more sense too."

Maya stood near the door. She had been with the team for the full two weeks this case had dragged on. She had watched Elias's presentations grow shorter each time — not from efficiency but from something closer to fatigue, the fatigue of a clinician who has ordered every reasonable test and still has nothing to offer a patient who is visibly suffering. She understood the fatigue. She was beginning to feel it herself.

Back in the workroom, Elias exhaled sharply. "He's inconsistent," he said. "The story keeps changing."

Maya looked up from her notes. "Or maybe we're missing something," she said. She said it the way she said most things — quietly, leaving room for it to be ignored if Elias needed it to be.

Elias did not respond. He returned to the chart.

The consults accumulated. Infectious disease. Rheumatology. Hematology. Each note ended the same way. Etiology unclear. Recommend continued workup. Elias felt the discomfort deepen each time another specialist failed to resolve it. The case had begun to feel, in some part of him he was not proud of, like a referendum on his own competence.

At the bedside again he found himself pressing harder than the moment required. "Are you sure about the timeline," he asked. "When exactly did the joint pain start, relative to the fevers."

The patient hesitated. "I think so," he said. "But it's hard to keep track, when it keeps moving around like this."

Elias nodded and wrote something down. He did not notice, in the moment, that what he wrote was not a new clinical thought.

Patient unable to provide consistent timeline.

It said nothing about the disease. It said something about the historian.

Maya saw the chart later that day. She read the line twice. She did not say anything to Elias. Not yet. She sat with a discomfort of her own.

She thought about the man with the chest pain. The story was true. Every part of it. She thought about the colon cancer case, the question she had learned to ask twice. This felt different. This was not a story that had been compressed into something too clean. This was a story that refused to compress at all, and the refusal itself was being treated as the patient's failure rather than as information.

That evening, she found Elias alone in the workroom.

"He said something to me today," she said, "when I sat with him for a few minutes after rounds." Elias looked up. "He said he feels like nobody believes him anymore. Not about being sick. About being honest."

Elias was quiet. "I didn't say that," he said.

He pulled up his note from two days earlier. Read it slowly. Patient unable to provide consistent timeline. He had not meant it as an accusation. He understood, reading it now, that meaning was not always what determined the effect.

He thought of the question he had been learning to carry — not what would make this not what I think it is, but something that fit this moment more precisely.

What would make this inconsistency not the patient's failure but the disease's truth.

He had been asking the question about the diagnosis. He had not been asking it about the patient. That was where the error lived.

The next morning a peripheral smear ordered almost as an afterthought by the hematology consultant returned with an answer. Abnormal cells. Hairy projections under the microscope.

Hairy cell leukemia. A rare indolent malignancy that infiltrates the spleen and bone marrow in a way that disrupts immune function without ever quite committing to a single dramatic presentation — producing instead exactly the kind of migratory, fluctuating, hard-to-pin-down symptoms that had frustrated everyone in this case for two full weeks.

The inconsistency had not been a flaw in the historian. It had been the disease, telling the truth in the only way it knew how.

That afternoon Elias sat with the patient to explain the diagnosis. "I want to apologize for something," he said, before he explained anything else.

The patient turned to him, surprised.

"There were moments," Elias said, "when I think you could tell I didn't quite believe how confusing this felt to you. I was frustrated that we couldn't find an answer. I let that frustration land somewhere it shouldn't have."

The patient was quiet. "I could tell," he said. Not unkindly. Simply honestly.

"It's a treatable disease," Elias said. "What you were describing the whole time was real. All of it. Even the parts that didn't fit together yet."

The patient nodded slowly. Something in his shoulders released slightly — in a way that had nothing to do with the prognosis and everything to do with finally being believed.

That night Elias wrote in his notebook.

When the story will not resolve, the irritation belongs to the case.
Do not let it find its way to the person telling it.
Ask what would make the inconsistency not the patient's failure
but the disease's truth.

Clinical Reflection

Cognitive dissonance arises when reality resists a clean explanation and the mind seeks relief — sometimes by dismissing the data, sometimes by reclassifying the patient from unwell to unreliable. The shift rarely announces itself; it arrives as a slightly sharper question, a note about consistency rather than symptoms, a change in tone the patient feels before the clinician notices it. But the inconsistency is not always a flaw in the historian. Some diseases produce migratory, contradictory pictures by their nature. There is a reliable warning that the question has stopped being asked: when a note begins describing the historian instead of the history, the reclassification has already happened. The discomfort belongs to the case, not to the person describing it.

PART II — CHAPTER 4

Authority Bias

The Voice That Ends the Discussion

When someone sounds certain,
thinking often stops.
Not because the answer is right.
But because it feels certain.
Some lessons are not taught.
They are survived.

The patient was admitted from clinic. Seventy-three years old. A history of prostate cancer, treated with radiation five years earlier. His initial presentation had shown locally invasive disease. His PSA had been climbing steadily. He had been losing weight. Abdominal fullness. Fatigue that his daughter said had crept up on him over the past two months.

Dr. Pierce was the patient's urologist: she knew the patient from years of visits in her clinic. She had called and arranged the direct admission.

By the time Elias received the admission the decision had already been made several steps above him.

"Given his history," Dr. Pierce said, "I think we have to assume this is the cancer progressing. I have been expecting this, based on his labs. At this stage, the kindest thing is to keep him comfortable."

The attending found Elias afterward. "No labs," she said. "No imaging. This is not a diagnostic admission. Comfort measures. I'll have the hospice consult placed first thing in the morning." She said it the way she said most things. Without inviting discussion.

Elias nodded. He wrote the orders.

Maya was with him that night. She had learned to read the stillness that came over Elias when something did not sit right and he had not yet decided what to do about it.

"He hasn't had any imaging since several months ago in the clinic," she said, reviewing the chart. "No recent labs either."

"The attending wants comfort measures," Elias said. He heard himself say it — the same flatness he had heard in his own voice before, on other cases, when a decision had been made above him and his job, as he understood it, was simply to carry it forward.

At the bedside, the patient was breathing a little fast. Uncomfortable. Not in obvious distress, but restless in the way of someone whose body is working harder than anyone in the room has acknowledged yet.

"It's my stomach," he told Elias. "Feels full all the time now. Hard to eat."

Elias examined him. His abdomen was full, distended, almost tense. A firm mass filling up his lower abdomen.

Elias sat with him. The room was quiet. The patient's breathing was fast. Not the breathing of a man whose body had made peace with what was happening to it.

He thought of the question he had been carrying. What would make this not cancer recurrence. He held it. The renal function had not been checked. The imaging had not been done. Nothing about the clinical picture explained a man who should have been declining and instead was breathing like someone whose body was working against an obstruction it could not name.

The question was there. The order above him had already answered it.

He ordered the labs anyway. He did not call the attending first.

The renal function returned severely abnormal. Not mildly elevated — the kind of number that belongs to an obstruction that has been building for days, quietly, while a room full of people agreed not to look.

He ordered a bedside ultrasound. Bilateral hydronephrosis — the dilated collecting systems visible on the screen like rivers backed up behind a dam. The bladder distended. Something obstructing both ureters. Possibly scarring from radiation. Possibly a mass. And the bladder was distended, filling up the lower abdominal cavity. Acute on chronic renal failure, building for days. Bladder outlet obstruction.

He called the attending. "I think this may not be cancer recurrence," he said. "The renal function is severely abnormal. Bilateral hydronephrosis and distended bladder on bedside ultrasound. I want to transfer him to the ICU and place a catheter tonight to see if this is reversible."

A pause on the line. "He has a history of metastatic disease," the attending said. "The kidneys failing is part of that process."

"We don't know that," Elias said. His voice was not steady.

"I have seen this before," the attending said. "Trust me on this one." The line was quiet. "Keep him comfortable. That's the order."

Elias did not argue further.

He did not yet understand, standing in the hallway with the phone still warm against his ear, that this moment — this exact moment — was the one he would return to for the rest of his life. Not the labs he had ordered. This. The choice not to push past a senior voice that sounded certain even though the evidence in front of both no longer supported certainty at all.

Maya stayed with him that night. Neither of them said very much. They sat with the patient as his breathing slowed. The daughter held his hand. Elias held the chart.

Somewhere in the space between those two things, a man died who might have had a different ending or might not have — they would never know which, because the question had never been allowed to fully ask itself.

Afterward in the workroom Elias did not speak for a long time. Maya sat across from him. She did not offer comfort yet. She understood, somehow, that comfort offered too early could quietly close something that needed to stay open a while longer.

"I knew something was wrong before I ordered the labs," Elias finally said. "I knew it the first night. I waited because the attending had already decided, and some part of me still believed that meant the deciding was no longer mine to do." He looked at his hands. "I don't know if it would have mattered. Maybe the cancer really had come back. Maybe nothing I did would have changed the ending. But I will never know that. And not knowing is so much worse than I thought it would be."

Lighthouse came in sometime after midnight. He was quiet.

"I had a patient once," he said.

That was all. Elias looked up.

"A long time ago," Lighthouse said. "Early in my training. I noticed something was wrong. I stood back longer than I should have. He died before I acted on what I knew." He did not say more than that. He let the sentence sit there, spare and unadorned, the way a person offers something not to be examined but simply to be known.

"I am not telling you this to make you feel less alone in the way you think," he said. "I am telling you because you are not as alone as you believe you are right now. That is different. And it matters."

He was quiet a moment. "Most physicians who practice long enough, and honestly enough, carry a small number of patients where something they did, or did not do, or allowed someone else to decide for them, changed how the story ended. Not negligence. Not malpractice. Just the ordinary, devastating weight of having been the variable at the exact moment it mattered most." He studied Elias. "Pretending that list does not exist is its own kind of harm."

He left.

Elias stood in the hallway a long while afterward. He thought of the question that had been there — present, formed, unanswered — while the voice on the phone carried the certainty of a senior physician who had seen enough to believe he was seeing this too.

The question could survive a label. It could survive a week of confident diagnoses. It had not survived that voice.

He would need to learn to make it louder than the voices that silenced it. He thought he might spend the rest of his career finding out.

That night he wrote in his notebook.

The question was there. I asked it, to myself,
The answer had already been given by someone whose voice
I did not know how to be louder than.
I will learn. I have to.

Clinical Reflection

Authority bias transfers the weight of a decision to whoever sounds most certain. It needs no wrong diagnosis and no careless physician — only a senior voice, a conclusion already reached, and a junior clinician who hasn't yet learned that the discomfort of disagreement is not evidence of being wrong. Its damage is precise: a finding surfaces that questions the accepted narrative, and instead of being answered it is absorbed, folded back into the story by the same certainty that built it. A question like that deserves to be asked aloud, where someone with the standing to be wrong must answer it. Asked quietly — to a chart, to oneself at midnight — it changes nothing except the asker, and the patient pays for the silence. The lesson is not that authority should never be trusted; most of the time the senior voice is right, which is exactly what makes the exceptions so hard to hear. It is that the discomfort of disagreement is not the same as being wrong. Sometimes it is the only evidence available that you are right — and the only thing standing between a patient and an ending no one intended.

PART II — CHAPTER 5

Groupthink

The Diagnosis Everyone Agreed On

When everyone agrees too quickly,
someone has stopped thinking.
Often, everyone.
Consensus feels like safety.
It is sometimes only company.

Five people agreed before noon. Every agreement sounded like evidence.

The patient was seventy-one years old. A retired letter carrier, half a pack of cigarettes a day for fifty years, an aspirin every morning since a cardiologist had prescribed one a decade earlier. He had fainted at home, at the kitchen table — his wife heard the chair go over from the next room. By the time the ambulance arrived he was awake, pale, and apologizing for the trouble. In the emergency department he described a deep ache low in his abdomen, hard to localize, present since just before he fell.

The pieces assembled themselves quickly. Acute anemia. Hemoglobin nine point one, down from twelve point three at his primary care office two months earlier. An ulcer history, back in his forties. The daily aspirin. A rectal exam with trace heme-positive stool. The emergency physician drafted the story in a single line: syncope secondary to acute blood loss anemia, likely upper GI source. It was a reasonable line. It explained the fall, the pallor, the hemoglobin, the stool. By the time the admission call was made, the sentence had done what well-made sentences do. It had become the case.

Elias presented him on rounds that morning. "Seventy-one-year-old male with syncope and acute on chronic anemia, heme-positive stool, on aspirin, with a remote ulcer history. GI bleed, likely upper source. GI is aware. NPO for endoscopy this afternoon, transfuse below seven, serial counts."

Maya, three months into her intern year, looked at the numbers and found nothing to disagree with. Daniel, beside her, said what she was thinking. "The aspirin plus the old ulcer. It writes itself." The GI fellow, reached by phone, listened to the summary, and agreed without coming to the bedside. "Sounds straightforward. Keep him comfortable, we'll scope him after the two o'clock." The plan was made. Every person who touched the case that morning arrived at the same conclusion, and each arrival made the next one easier, the way footprints make a path.

Nobody in the room was deferring to anybody. That was what none of them could see. There was no senior voice overriding a junior one, no reluctant silence, no doubt swallowed for the sake of hierarchy. There was only agreement, freely given, five times over — and a room in which the question what else could this be had died of unanimity, because a question needs at least one person who feels it, and the agreement had made the room feel finished.

At the bedside, the patient shifted against the gurney, trying to find a position that solved the ache.

"You're sure it's my stomach," he said. "It doesn't feel like my stomach. It feels lower. And it goes through to my back."

"The gurneys do that to everyone," the nurse said kindly, adjusting his pillow. She was not wrong about the gurneys.

"It started before I fell, though," he said. But the room had moved on to the consent forms, and he was a polite man, and he let it go.

Maya charted the exchange. Patient reports lower abdominal discomfort radiating to back, likely positional. The word likely did the quiet work such words do. His morning chemistries sat in the chart alongside the note — BUN fourteen, creatinine normal, a ratio that had nothing to say in favor of a large gastrointestinal bleed and was asked no questions. His abdomen was soft, obese, mildly and vaguely tender. Nobody was feeling for a mass because nobody was looking for one. In fifty years of smoking no one had ever put an ultrasound probe on his aorta. There had never been a reason. There was, that morning, still not felt to be one.

The endoscopy was performed at three. The stomach was clean. The duodenum was clean. Old scarring in the bulb, healed, undisturbed. No blood, no ulcer, no source.

The negative scope arrived in a room that had spent the entire day agreeing, and the room did with it what rooms in that condition do. It did not reopen the question. It rescheduled it. "Must be lower," the fellow said, snapping off his gloves. "We'll prep him tonight and do a colonoscopy in the morning." Heads nodded. It was not an unreasonable next step. It was simply the only kind of step still available to a diagnosis that had stopped being a hypothesis and become the premise — the thing new evidence was interpreted within rather than evaluated against. The scope that found nothing had been sent to find a bleed. Not finding one, it was assumed to have looked in the wrong place. Nobody said aloud, or thought, that it might have been sent for the wrong thing entirely.

The patient started the prep solution at seven. At nine-forty, the nurse found him gray and slick with sweat, his pressure seventy over palp, his eyes rolling as she reached him. The crash response arrived within two minutes. Fluids ran wide. And a resident from the ICU team, working through the causes of unexplained collapse in the order she had been trained to, put an ultrasound probe on his abdomen.

The aorta filled the screen. Seven point eight centimeters where two would have been normal, and along its left flank a dark smear that had no business being there.

The ache in his back, the syncope at the kitchen table, the falling hemoglobin — all of it had been the aneurysm, leaking slowly, contained by nothing more than tissue and luck, for something over a day. The sixty-second scan that found it had been available since the moment he arrived.

Vascular surgery had him in the operating room within forty minutes. The leak had ruptured freely, but recently; the repair was long, the transfusions many. He survived — the vascular surgeon, closing, put it plainly: an hour later, and this is a different conversation. He spent nine days in the ICU. The trace of blood in his stool was traced, eventually, to hemorrhoids, and to an aspirin doing exactly what aspirin does. It had never had anything to do with anything.

The workroom that night was quiet in the way rooms are quiet after luck has been the difference.

"I keep going back through the day," Maya said, "looking for the moment I saw something and didn't say it. The moment I stayed quiet." She shook her head slowly. "It isn't there. I never had the doubt. I agreed. It felt like being part of a team."

"It was," Lighthouse said from the doorway. He came in and sat. "That is what makes this one treacherous. The other failures cost you something — overruling your doubt, deferring to a voice, pushing past your own fatigue. This one feels like collegiality while it is happening. It feels like the thing we ask of you."

He watched Elias. "Who disagreed with the diagnosis this morning."

"No one," Elias said.

"That was the problem," Lighthouse said. "Five people agreed. It felt like five reasons. It was one reason — a well-made sentence in an emergency department note — repeated five times by five people, each of whom heard the others' agreement as confirmation. Confirmation requires independence. There was none in that room. There was one judgment, echoed."

He was quiet. "There were questions available all day, waiting for a single doubter to pick them up. A bleed that drops a man to the floor leaves a trail — vomit, melena, hematochezia, something. Usually a lot. Where was the blood. Nobody asked, because the room had answered. His chemistry never believed the diagnosis. The BUN should rise if there is blood in the GI tract. He told you himself the pain was lower, and went through to his back, and had started before he fell." He looked at both of them. "And then the scope came back clean, and the diagnosis survived it. That is the finding I want you to remember from tonight. Not the aneurysm. The scheduling. A test that should have broken the agreement was converted into an appointment for tomorrow."

"How do you defend against something nobody feels happening," Maya asked.

"You stop relying on someone feeling it," Lighthouse said. "Courage is a poor system. Before a room closes a diagnosis, one person — any person, assigned out loud — states the best case against it. Not doubts. The best case. If the best case against is weak, you have lost two minutes. If no one can be found to make it, that is not evidence the diagnosis is right." He stood. "Five people agreed this morning. Not one of them argued the other side. That is not five examinations of the diagnosis. It is one diagnosis, looked at once and approved five times."

That night, Maya wrote in her notebook.

Agreement felt like teamwork,
all the way to the operating room.
Next time a room agrees this easily,
someone must be assigned to argue against it.
It might as well be me.

Elias, in his own notebook, wrote:

Five of us agreed.
It was one reason, said five times.
The clean scope should have ended the diagnosis.
We gave it a new appointment instead.
Where was the blood —
one question, all day,
and nobody's job to ask it.

Clinical Reflection

Groupthink is not authority bias — no senior voice silences a junior one — and not momentum. It is convergence in real time among peers: agreement functioning as verification. Five clinicians concurring feels like five separate examinations reaching one result, when it is often one framing, absorbed early and echoed until the echoes are mistaken for a chorus. It is pleasant, which is why no one inside it can point to a moment of suppression. Its signature: disconfirming evidence stops reopening questions and starts generating logistics — a surprising negative rerouted into another study, another appointment. When your first move after a surprise is to schedule something rather than reconsider something, the room has closed. So before a diagnosis closes, assign one person, aloud, to argue the best case against it. Consensus never opposed is not a verdict.

PART II — CHAPTER 6

Cognitive Ease

The Shortcut Everyone Took

What feels easy often feels right.
The mind prefers fluency to friction.
Familiarity is not the same as understanding.

The admission was routine. That made it seem easier.

The patient was seventy-two years old, a Navy veteran, a fact he carried proudly on the cap he wore everywhere he went: USS Kitty Hawk, CV-63. Cough. Low-grade fever. Shortness of breath. He had been admitted twice before in the past year with the same symptoms, the same chest X-ray pattern, the same diagnosis. Recurrent pneumonia, right lower lobe, responding each time to a standard course of antibiotics.

On rounds, Elias presented briskly. "Seventy-two-year-old male Navy veteran with recurrent right lower lobe pneumonia. Presentation consistent with prior two admissions. Starting the same antibiotic regimen that's worked before."

No one objected. The pattern was familiar enough that objecting would have required a reason nobody in the room felt compelled to find.

A CT chest was ordered, mostly as due diligence, given that this was his third admission in under a year for the same complaint. The read came back unremarkable. Findings consistent with post-infectious changes, right lower lobe. No mass identified. The radiologist who read it was working through a heavy list that day, on a study that was not, technically, optimized for central airway evaluation, and did not catch what was sitting just proximal to where everyone's attention was already focused. The negative CT did something almost worse than no CT at all. It closed the question.

At the bedside, the patient spoke softly. "Feels just like the last two times," he said. "I figured this was coming, eventually. Seems to happen every few months now." Elias nodded. He had heard this before, almost word for word, on the two previous admissions, documented in two previous notes that this note was beginning to resemble closely enough that copying forward would have changed very little.

Maya reviewed the chart that afternoon. She noticed the CT read. Unremarkable. She noticed, too, something in the nursing flow sheet that nobody had flagged. His oxygen saturation dropped several points each time he sat upright, then recovered somewhat when he reclined.

"That's a little unusual for pneumonia," she said to Elias in the workroom.

"It happens," Elias said. "Positional changes can cause the perfusion and oxygenation of the lung to be mismatched. Especially with this much right lower lobe involvement."

It was not an unreasonable answer. It was also not one he had taken the time to fully interrogate before offering it. Maya let it go, for the moment, though she wrote it down in her own notes — the habit she had built over the past several months of keeping a private record of things that did not yet have anywhere else to live.

The antibiotics continued. The pattern held, the way familiar patterns do, each day's presentation echoing the day before it closely enough that nobody felt the pull to look again with fresh eyes. This had happened before. It would resolve again the way it had resolved before. That belief, reasonable on its surface, had taken on a momentum of its own.

Three days into the admission, in the early evening, Maya was at the bedside rechecking his lung exam, and a nurse was adjusting his IV when he began to cough. Hard, then harder. Blood. A significant amount, arriving fast, the patient's eyes widening with the fear of someone whose body has just told him something no one had warned him to expect. Maya did not hesitate. She hit the call button, turned him onto his side, and called for help in a voice that brought two nurses and a resident into the room within seconds.

Elias arrived moments later. The bleeding was significant. Not yet life-threatening but moving in a direction that left no room for the comfortable pace of the past three days. He did not wait for imaging. He did not wait for a formal consult request to wind through the usual channels. He picked up the phone himself and called the pulmonary fellow on call, his voice clear and fast. "I need emergent bronchoscopy. Massive hemoptysis. Recurrent pneumonia, same lobe, three admissions in under a year. I think we missed something."

The bronchoscopy was performed within the hour. The pulmonologist found it almost immediately. A mass, paratracheal, extending into the proximal airway, positioned in exactly the location a standard chest CT, read for parenchymal findings rather than central airway anatomy, would plausibly miss. It had been narrowing his airway slowly, for months, creating the exact post-obstructive pattern that had been diagnosed, three times now, as ordinary recurrent pneumonia. Biopsies were taken. The pathology, when it returned, showed adenocarcinoma — the kind sometimes associated, the oncologist later explained, with prolonged occupational exposure to asbestos, the kind of exposure common among Navy personnel of his generation, serving on ships insulated with materials nobody understood the danger of at the time. He had carried it, unknowingly, since long before anyone in that room had been born.

Elias went back to the bedside that evening, before the oncology team's formal visit. The man was sitting up, the cap on the tray table beside him.

"The pneumonia was real," Elias said. "All three times. But it kept happening in the same place for a reason. There's a growth beside the main airway on the right side, and it has been slowly narrowing the passage — like a branch fallen across a stream. The part of the lung behind it can't drain or clear itself. So infection keeps settling there. We treat it, it clears, the blockage stays, and it comes back."

The man absorbed this with the steadiness of someone who had spent a career on machinery. "So, you fix the blockage," he said, "or you keep bailing water."

"That's exactly right," Elias said. "We can remove the obstruction, but this is lung cancer. We will have to wait and see how this goes from here. Fixing the obstruction is only the first part."

That evening, in the workroom, Elias sat across from Maya.

"You noticed the oxygen dropping," he said. "Before any of this."

"I did," Maya said.

"You had an explanation for it," she corrected gently. "I wrote it down and let it go."

"It wasn't wrong, exactly," Elias said. "Positional V/Q changes happen. It just wasn't the only possible explanation, and I didn't bother chasing the other ones." He looked at the CT report, still open on the screen. "Three admissions. Same diagnosis, three times. A negative CT that I let close the question instead of just narrowing it."

Lighthouse appeared in the doorway. He studied the imaging.

"Familiarity is its own kind of sedative," he said. He sat down. "The first admission, you investigate carefully. The second, a little less. By the third, the pattern itself has started doing the thinking for you." He looked at Elias. "The CT did not help you here. Not because it was wrong to order. Because a reassuring scan, layered on top of an already familiar story, made the question feel more closed than it actually was."

Maya spoke quietly. "I had a different explanation in my notes. I didn't push it very hard."

"Why not," Lighthouse asked.

She considered this honestly. "Because Elias had an answer that made sense. And it was easier to write something down than to keep asking after someone more experienced than me had already responded."

Lighthouse nodded. "Cognitive ease moves in both directions," he said. "It is not only the clinician who stops working harder once a pattern feels familiar. It is also the learner who accepts an explanation because it arrived quickly, and confidently, from someone she trusted." He looked between them. "The mass is currently being addressed. The bleeding is controlled. This is not the worst version of this story. The cancer will have its own trajectory. But this could have been caught on the first admission, or the second, and familiarity made the third one feel like nothing new was required."

That night, Elias wrote in his notebook.

The story being the same does not mean the cause is.
A reassuring test does not end a question.
It only answers the part it was designed to ask.

Maya, in her own notebook, wrote something shorter.

An answer that arrives quickly
deserves the same scrutiny as one that arrives slowly.
Even when I trust the person giving it to me.

Clinical Reflection

Cognitive ease is not laziness. It is the mind doing what minds are built to do — recognizing a pattern and trusting it a little more each time it repeats. Fluency feels like accuracy: an explanation that arrives quickly, without friction, carries a sense of rightness that has nothing to do with whether it is right. The feeling is a property of the processing, not of the world. The antidote is not distrust of every familiar pattern — that is most of what expertise is. It is a single habit: when a story repeats for the third time, ask what a first encounter would require of you, and provide it again. Mistaking ease for evidence is the danger, not the ease itself.

PART II — CHAPTER 7

Normalization of Deviance

The Exception Everyone Stopped Noticing

When something goes wrong often enough,
it stops feeling wrong.
It becomes familiar.
Then acceptable.
Then invisible.

The abnormal lab was not new. By now it was accepted as his new normal.

The patient was sixty-nine years old. Chronic kidney disease, diabetes, hypertension. He had been admitted many times before, often enough that the nursing staff greeted him by name, and the chart itself had the thickness of a life that medicine had been tracking closely for a very long time. His potassium was elevated. Five point eight. Not dramatically. Not urgently, on its face. Just enough to notice.

Maya reviewed his labs that morning with Daniel, the two of them moving through a stack of patients together the way interns on the same service often did — comparing notes, thinking out loud, in the shorthand that develops between people learning the same things at the same time.

"His potassium's up a little," she said. "Five-eight."

Daniel glanced at the prior values. "He runs high, though. Look — five-four last admission. Five-six the one before that."

Maya watched the trend. He was right. The number had been elevated, in some degree, on each of his last several admissions. It had never, in that time, caused a problem.

"Probably just his baseline," she said.

"Probably," Daniel agreed.

Neither of them mentioned it on rounds that morning. Not because they had decided, consciously, that it did not matter. Because it had stopped registering, between them, as something that required a decision at all. The number fit a pattern they had both, independently and then together, absorbed as simply who this patient was. A man who ran a little high. Always had, as far as either of them had ever seen.

Elias was on a different part of the service that day, absorbed in two new admissions that had come in back-to-back, unaware that the conversation between Maya and Daniel had even taken place. He was not in the room for it. He would not have known to ask. The potassium did not appear in the morning presentation because neither intern had flagged it as something worth presenting. It was simply there, in the chart, the way it had always been there, on every admission anyone could remember.

At the bedside, the patient mentioned it himself, almost as an aside, to the nurse drawing his afternoon labs. "They always tell me it's a little high," he said. "Never seems to matter much." He said it without concern. He had been told this enough times, by enough people, across enough admissions, that his own instinct to worry had been worn down to something closer to resignation. If it had mattered, someone would have said so. Nobody had. So it must not.

The afternoon labs were not drawn until early evening, delayed behind several other patients on a busy floor. When they returned, his potassium was six point three. The result populated in the system at nine forty-seven p.m. Nobody saw it immediately. The night team was occupied with two new admissions of their own, and the lab, without a clinician actively watching for it, sat in the chart the way results sometimes do on the busiest nights, waiting to be noticed rather than surfacing itself.

Maya was on call that night. She did not check his labs again before midnight. She had seen the morning value. She had already decided that hours earlier, in the kind of decision that does not feel like a decision at the time it is made, that this was simply how he ran.

At eleven-twenty p.m., the monitor alarmed. Ventricular tachycardia, degenerating quickly. The code team arrived within minutes. Maya was among the first in the room, running the code alongside the senior resident on call, her body doing exactly what it had been trained to do while some other part of her mind was already, faintly, beginning to understand what this was going to mean once it was over. The potassium, redrawn during the code, came back at seven point one. The arrhythmia resolved after calcium, insulin, and dextrose, and emergent dialysis was arranged within the hour. He survived. Barely, and not without a difficult several days that followed.

Maya did not sleep that night. She sat in the workroom long after the code had ended, the chart open in front of her, scrolling back through every potassium value across every admission she could find. Five-four. Five-six. Five-eight. Six-three. Seven-one. A slow climb, visible only now, in retrospect, as a climb at all. At the time, each individual number had simply looked like the one before it.

Elias found her there just after six in the morning. He had heard about the code the moment he arrived. He did not ask her to walk him through it right away. He sat down across from her.

"You were in the room. You've been carrying it since," Elias said. He glanced at the chart open in front of her. "I'm not here to add to that."

"I know," Maya said.

"I'm not asking because I think it should have come to me. I'm asking because I want to understand what happened."

Maya didn't answer at first. "Daniel and I looked at the trend together," she said. "It had been high before. Several times. Nothing had ever happened. We decided it was just his baseline, and we didn't think about it again." She looked at the screen, at the five numbers, climbing. "I didn't get it wrong because someone told me not to worry. I got it wrong because I told myself not to worry, and I had a colleague who agreed with me, and that agreement felt like enough."

Lighthouse arrived a short while later, having heard, the way he always seemed to hear, about the codes that happened overnight. He did not ask what went wrong. He had already seen the trend.

"How many admissions," he asked, "before a number like this stops feeling like a number and starts feeling like a fact about a person."

Maya considered the question honestly. "I'm not sure. Three, maybe. This was his fourth."

Lighthouse took that in. "Normalization of deviance rarely involves a single decision," he said. "It involves several small ones, each reasonable in isolation, accumulating into something nobody quite decided on purpose." He looked at her. "You were not negligent. You were precisely as careful as the pattern allowed you to be. That is the danger. The pattern itself becomes the argument against vigilance."

Maya thought of Daniel, agreeing with her that morning, the two of them arriving at the same comfortable conclusion independently enough that neither had felt the friction that might have stopped them.

"It wasn't just me," she said.

"No," Lighthouse said. "It rarely is. Deviance normalizes faster when it is shared. Two people agreeing feels like confirmation. It is sometimes only two people making the same mistake at the same time, and mistaking that for consensus."

That morning, Maya found Daniel in the workroom. She told him what had happened overnight. He was quiet.

"We both studied the same numbers," he said. "We both decided they didn't mean anything."

"We did," Maya said.

"I keep thinking that if it had been just me, alone, looking at that trend, I might have felt less certain. Having someone else agree made it feel confirmed."

Maya nodded. "I think that's exactly what happened."

That night, Maya wrote in her notebook.

Two people agreeing is not two people analyzing.
Recheck the one thing that has stopped feeling abnormal.
That is exactly when it is most worth repeating.

Clinical Reflection

Normalization of deviance requires only repetition and the comfort it provides. An abnormal finding is noticed once, noted the second time, and by the third or fourth has become descriptive rather than diagnostic — no longer a warning, simply a trait. Each judgment along the way is defensible; the danger lives in the accumulation, where no single encounter is wrong and the sum is fatal. Two clinicians can reach the same comfortable conclusion independently and mistake each other's agreement for a second opinion neither earned. Aim the discipline exactly at the findings that have stopped feeling alarming: when an abnormality has been seen before, without consequence, ask what would have to be true for this time to be different. Then check whether it already is.

PART II — CHAPTER 8

Protocol Fixation

The Patient Who Did Not Fit the Protocol

Protocols are maps.
They are not the terrain.
When the patient diverges,
the map must be questioned.
Sometimes it is questioned too late.

He collapsed at the end of the meal. That detail mattered later, though no one quite understood how much at the time.

A private dining room, in one of the city's most exclusive steakhouses, the kind of place where the staff knew his name before he gave it. He was sixty-one. Prominent. The kind of man whose collapse generated a phone call before the ambulance had even arrived, because someone at the table knew exactly who to call.

Dr. Thomas, the chief of cardiology, took that call directly. He knew the patient. Not as a physician knows a patient — as a friend knows a friend. Forty years, give or take. College, fraternity brothers, golf, then life. The kind of friendship that makes a man answer his phone at any hour without exception. He came in himself and met him at the door of the emergency department.

"Chest pain," the patient managed, between labored breaths. "Started right after dinner. Severe."

Diaphoretic. Tachycardic. The presentation, on its surface, fit precisely.

Dr. Thomas initiated the ACS protocol himself, standing at the bedside, with the fluency of someone who had run this protocol hundreds of times and trusted it completely. EKG. Troponin, first draw. Aspirin. Oxygen. The orders moved through the system the way they were designed to, each step prompting the next, the protocol functioning exactly as it had been built to function.

"I have a meeting I can't move," Dr. Thomas told the resident on duty. "A call with a hospital in Japan. It has been scheduled for months. Run the protocol. Page me with the troponin."

He left within the hour. He did not think, leaving, that he was leaving anything unfinished. The protocol was running. That was, in his understanding, the same as the patient being taken care of.

Elias and Maya came on for the night shift partway through the workup, picking up a service that was, by then, simply executing a plan already in motion.

"Sixty-one-year-old male, acute chest pain and diaphoresis following a meal," the day resident told them at sign-out. "ACS protocol initiated by Dr. Thomas. First troponin pending."

Elias reviewed the chart. Nothing about it prompted him to question what was already underway. Nothing prompted him to reexamine the patient. A respected cardiologist had seen the patient himself, at the bedside, and started the workup personally. That carried its own weight.

At the bedside, the patient spoke, quieter now, the diaphoresis still present but the acute distress somewhat eased by the oxygen and the reassurance of a room full of people clearly working hard on his behalf. "This pain is different," he said. "Sharper than I expected. And it hurts more when I swallow."

Maya was charting nearby. She heard it. She wrote it down, the way she had learned to write things down, though in the moment it did not register as something that broke from the picture already forming. Chest pain. Diaphoresis. A cardiologist's initial impression. The detail about swallowing sat in her note without yet finding anywhere else to live.

The first troponin returned negative. Within normal limits. This did not rule out ACS — the protocol accounted for that, calling for a second troponin several hours later, the standard interval built into the algorithm for exactly this reason. The team continued forward. Pain medication for comfort. Continued monitoring. The plan, as written, was sound. It was also, by then, the only plan anyone was actively considering.

The second troponin, when it returned, was also negative. On paper, this was reassuring. The patient remained uncomfortable. Not improving the way a resolving cardiac event typically would, but not acutely worse, either. The protocol had no next step designed for a patient who was simply, persistently, uncomfortable in a way that did not fit neatly into either column.

The call came to Lighthouse just before midnight. Dr. Thomas himself.

"I need you to look at something," he said. "A patient of mine. A friend, actually. Something isn't right and I can't put my finger on it. I've already started the ACS protocol. Everything is running. But it's not —" He paused. "Would you go in and look at him. A favor to me."

Lighthouse came.

He stood at the bedside before touching the patient at all. He listened to the story, unfiltered by the hours that had already organized it into an ACS narrative.

"Tell me about the pain again," he said. "From the beginning."

The patient, exhausted now, told it again. The meal. A large one. Wine. Then, near the end, a sudden urge to vomit, which he had managed, briefly, in the restroom, before the pain began in earnest. He had not mentioned the vomiting before. No one had asked. The protocol's questions had all pointed toward the heart. None of them had asked about the meal, or what had happened right before the pain started.

Lighthouse examined his neck, then his upper chest. Pressed gently. A faint crackling beneath his fingers. Subcutaneous emphysema. Air where air did not belong, trapped beneath the skin, the unmistakable signature of a process that had nothing to do with the heart at all.

"I need a CT of the chest immediately," Lighthouse said, his voice still quiet but carrying a different weight now. "With oral contrast, if he can tolerate it. I think this is an esophageal rupture."

The room, which had spent six hours moving through a single, well-worn path, turned all at once.

The CT confirmed it. A tear in the distal esophagus. Mediastinal air, extensive. Early signs of mediastinitis already visible, the infection spreading into the space between the lungs with the speed that makes this injury one of the most lethal in all of surgery. Boerhaave syndrome. Forceful vomiting, against a closed airway, rupturing the esophageal wall under pressure it was never built to withstand.

Cardiothoracic surgery was called emergently. The patient was taken to the operating room within the hour. The delay, by then, was measured in many hours, not minutes — time during which gastric contents and oral bacteria had been spreading through his mediastinum, seeding an infection that surgery alone, however urgently performed, could not fully outrun.

He would not survive it. The dying took eight days — overwhelming mediastinitis, then septic shock, then the slow cascade of multi-organ failure that the surgery and the antibiotics could slow but never outrun.

Dr. Thomas returned the following morning, having heard only partially what had happened overnight. He stood in the hallway outside the surgical ICU for a long time. He did not speak to anyone right away.

Elias found Maya in the workroom later that day. Neither of them said much at first.

"He told us the pain was different," Maya finally said. "He said it hurt to swallow. I wrote it down. I didn't say it out loud."

"Neither did I," Elias said. "I read your note. I didn't follow up on it either." He looked at the chart, still open, the protocol's steps laid out cleanly, each box checked in precisely the order it was designed to be checked. "The protocol worked exactly the way it was supposed to work. That's what makes this hard to look at. Nobody did anything wrong, by the protocol's own measure. The protocol just wasn't built to ask about swallowing."

Lighthouse came in quietly. He did not sit right away.

"I want to say something," he said, "and I want you to hear it clearly. The protocol is not the failure here. The protocol does exactly what it was designed to do — it catches a great many heart attacks quickly and reliably. The failure is in treating the protocol as a complete examination, rather than as one tool among several." He watched both of them. "He told you the pain was different. Twice, by my reading of the chart. Once to the nurse. Once to you." He paused. "A protocol cannot listen. Only the people running it can."

Maya did not write a clinical pearl that night. She wrote a single thought and did not add anything beneath it.

He told us.
I wrote it down.
A checklist is not the same as listening.

Elias, in his own notebook, wrote something he did not show anyone.

Some patients do not survive
the time it takes a protocol to ask the right question.
I will not forget what his voice sounded like
when he said the pain was different.

He closed the notebook. He did not open it again for several days.

Clinical Reflection

Protocols save lives, reliably and at scale, in moments when individual judgment would be too slow. But every protocol is narrow by design: it asks the questions its target diagnosis requires and no others, and information outside those questions has nowhere to go. A protocol running smoothly generates its own reassurance — boxes checked, intervals honored — that can substitute for anyone re-examining the premise. The antidote is a single habit, kept regardless of who launched the pathway: a patient's statement that this is different is data of a specific kind, a comparison across time no algorithm can make. When a patient says this is different, stop, and ask what the protocol was never built to ask. Even when every box is checked. Especially then.

PART II — CHAPTER 9

Moral Disengagement

The Case That Felt Smaller

Some cases fail not because they are difficult,
but because no one believes they are important.
The patient knows.
She always knows.

Her name was Rena.

She had been a hospital aide once, twenty years earlier, before a divorce and a back injury and a slow unraveling that she could describe, when asked, with more clarity and self-awareness than most people brought to their own simpler lives. She had been homeless for six years. Alcohol use disorder, chronic pain from the old injury, a chart thick enough that opening it took a moment longer than opening most. She came to this hospital often. The nurses knew her by name. They knew her favorite snacks and kept them on hand — an orange soda and cheese crackers. The residents knew her name too. But knowing her name and knowing her had become, somewhere along the way, two different things.

She arrived that evening on her own, walking in slowly, holding the doorframe before letting go.

"I just don't feel right," she told the triage nurse. "Weak. Dizzy. Hard to explain."

It was, on its surface, a vague complaint. It was also, for Rena specifically, not an unfamiliar one. She had presented with versions of this same sentence many times before, and most of those times the explanation had been straightforward. Dehydration. Early withdrawal. A body that had been asked to carry too much, for too long, without enough support.

Elias picked up her chart between two other admissions. He had seen her before, more than once, though he could not have said, if asked directly, how many times exactly. On rounds, he presented her briefly. "Forty-seven-year-old female, known history of alcohol use disorder and chronic pain, presenting with nonspecific weakness and dizziness. Vitals stable. Likely dehydration, possible early withdrawal. Plan for fluids and monitoring."

The presentation took less time than the others that morning. No one in the room noticed this, including Elias. It simply moved faster, the way familiar things do.

At the bedside, Rena sat on the edge of the gurney, her hands folded carefully in her lap.

"I feel different this time," she said. She said it. Not dramatically. The quiet of someone who has learned, over many admissions, that saying things too forcefully rarely changed how quickly they were addressed.

Elias nodded. He did not sit down. "We'll get you some fluids," he said. "That usually helps."

Maya stood near the door, chart in hand, watching the exchange the way she had learned to watch things that did not yet have a name. She noticed Rena's eyes, slightly slower to track than they had seemed on the last admission several weeks earlier — an admission Maya happened to remember because she had been the intern admitting her that time too.

"She seems a little more confused than I remember," Maya said, once they were back in the hallway.

"Her baseline's hard to pin down," Elias said. "With the alcohol use, it varies."

It was not an unreasonable answer. It was also, Maya noticed without yet having words for the feeling, an answer that closed the question rather than opening it.

The labs were ordered. Not urgently. They sat in the queue behind labs for patients whose presentations had generated more immediate concern — the unspoken triage that happens not at the official level of acuity but in the quieter calculus of which patient a busy team decides to chase. The imaging that might have been ordered in another patient, on the strength of vague neurological complaints in someone with a fall risk and a bleeding risk from chronic alcohol use, was not ordered at all. Nobody decided against it, exactly. Nobody decided anything. The case simply moved at the pace the team had unconsciously assigned it.

Maya sat with Rena for a few minutes that afternoon, between other tasks, the way she had started doing with patients whose charts felt thinner than their lives were.

"Can you tell me more about what feels different," Maya asked.

Rena considered the question carefully, the way a person does when someone has finally asked it as though they wanted the real answer.

"I worked in a hospital once," she said. "Long time ago. I know what it's like when people think they already know your story before you finish telling it." She looked at Maya. "You're actually listening. I can tell the difference."

Maya felt something tighten in her chest. "What does different feel like," she asked again, gently.

"Heavier," Rena said. "On one side. Like my head doesn't quite agree with the rest of me."

Maya wrote this down carefully. She brought it to Elias.

"She says it's worse on one side," Maya said. "She used the word heavier. I don't think this is just withdrawal or dehydration."

Elias looked up from another chart. He was tired. The service was full. Rena's vitals, on the monitor, remained stable — the number that, in a busy department, often did more talking than anything a patient said out loud.

"Let's get a CT," he said. "Just to be safe."

It was the right call. It was also, Maya noticed, delivered with less urgency than he might have used for a different patient with the same words in her chart.

The order went in. It did not move quickly. The department was busy. Rena was stable. The particular invisible sorting that determines which stable patient gets scanned in twenty minutes and which gets scanned in three hours worked, that evening, the way it often worked for patients like her — not through any single decision, but through the accumulated weight of a hundred small assumptions about how much urgency her case actually deserved.

She fell just after seven that evening, attempting to walk to the bathroom without calling for help, the way she had learned, over many admissions, not to ask for things she suspected would take too long to arrive. A nurse found her on the floor. Conscious, but more confused now, one pupil sluggish in a way the other was not. The CT, finally performed emergently, showed a subdural hematoma, significant, with early midline shift. Neurosurgery was called immediately.

The evacuation was done urgently, unlike everything else in this case. The recovery was difficult, complicated by the alcohol use disorder that had, ironically, both contributed to her fall risk and made her chronic, low-grade confusion seem unremarkable enough to delay the imaging that ultimately saved her. She remained hospitalized for nearly three weeks. She went, eventually, to a rehabilitation facility, then to transitional housing arranged through social work — a slightly different ending than the one her chart's familiar thinness had seemed to be writing for her.

That night, in the workroom, Elias sat a long while without speaking. Maya sat across from him.

"I ordered the CT," he finally said. "I want to feel like that means something. But I ordered it slower than I would have for someone else." He turned to Maya. "You knew before I did. You sat with her. I didn't."

"I didn't push hard enough either," Maya said. "I told you what she said. I didn't tell you how much it mattered to me that nobody else had stopped to ask her."

By now it was early morning. Lighthouse arrived just before report. He did not ask what had happened clinically. He had already read the chart.

"Why do you think this case felt smaller," he asked.

Elias considered the question honestly. "Because she's been here so many times. Because the story always sounded the same. I think some part of me had already decided what this admission was before I walked in the room."

Lighthouse nodded. "Moral disengagement doesn't require disliking a patient," he said. "It requires only familiarity, and the particular fatigue that comes from caring fully, every time, for people whose lives keep bringing them back to the same difficult place." He looked at them. "She is not a different category of patient. She is a patient whose case has been made to feel smaller, by every encounter that treated her as familiar rather than as new."

"She told me she could tell I was actually listening," Maya said quietly. "As if that was unusual enough to be worth saying out loud."

Lighthouse didn't respond right away. "That should not be remarkable," he said. "The fact that it was, for her, is the entire lesson."

That night, Maya wrote in her notebook.

She knew the difference
between being seen and being processed.
I want every patient to be able to tell
which one they're getting.

Elias, in his own notebook, wrote something he sat with a while before closing the book.

Familiarity is not the same as understanding.
A patient who returns often is not asking less of you.
It is your job to make sure that is not what they receive.

Clinical Reflection

Moral disengagement rarely announces itself as indifference. It arrives disguised as familiarity — the fatigue of caring for patients who return again and again without the resources to break the pattern. No one decides to care less; the caring simply gets rationed, encounter by encounter, by a triage that appears in no order set. A history of benign admissions works like a prior probability — a legitimate tool — until the prior stops adjusting, hardens into an identity, and new information is absorbed into the old story rather than tested against it. The antidote is not extraordinary effort for certain patients. It is the refusal to let any case feel smaller because its story has become familiar. Every admission deserves the first one's workup — because the disease doesn't know it isn't the first.

PART II — CHAPTER 10

Diffusion of Responsibility

The Decision No One Owned

When everyone is involved,
no one feels responsible.
Decisions blur.
Ownership disappears.
Someone must decide.
And say so.

The plan had not moved forward. The way plans get buried in multiple consults.

The patient was sixty-four years old. Shortness of breath. Hypoxia. Borderline blood pressure. The case was complex, genuinely complex, in the way that does not resolve into a single clean diagnosis no matter how carefully it is examined. Pulmonary. Cardiac. Renal. Each system contributing, each system complicating what the others were trying to do.

On rounds that morning, Elias presented carefully. "Sixty-four-year-old male with multifactorial respiratory failure. Pulmonary, cardiology, and nephrology all involved. Plan under discussion."

The words sounded thorough. They were, Maya thought, listening from beside him, also strangely empty. A plan under discussion was not, in itself, a plan.

At the bedside, the patient was on four liters by nasal cannula, working visibly, each breath requiring more effort than the one before it.

"Am I getting better," he asked, between breaths.

Elias hesitated. "We're watching closely," he said.

It was true. It was also not an answer to the question the patient had asked.

The consultants weighed in over the course of the morning, each one thorough, each one reasonable, each one speaking only to the piece of the patient that belonged to their own expertise. Pulmonary recommended diuresis, to relieve the fluid contributing to his hypoxia. Cardiology advised caution, concerned that aggressive diuresis, in a patient with his blood pressure, risked underperfusing an already strained heart. Nephrology — Dr. Cynthia Evans, whose notes had a reputation on the house staff for being the most thorough and insightful in the building — recommended delay, noting that his kidney function could not safely tolerate rapid fluid shifts in either direction.

Each recommendation, read individually, was sound. Together, they canceled each other out almost entirely.

By early afternoon, the four liters had become six. The patient had stopped finishing his sentences. His blood gas, redrawn at two, was worse than the morning's — not dramatically, but moving, the way numbers move when a process has stopped waiting for the people managing it. The respiratory therapist mentioned high-flow. Nobody ordered it yet. Nobody ordered anything. The three consult notes sat in the chart, unreconciled, each one internally complete, each one waiting for someone else to act on it.

Maya reviewed them side by side in the workroom.

"So, what are we doing," she said, to no one, though Elias was the only one in the room to hear it.

It was not quite a complaint. It was closer to the plainest possible question, asked because she genuinely did not know the answer, and suspected, watching the three notes sit there, that no one else did either.

Elias studied the screen. He thought, briefly, of a man at a steakhouse who had said the pain was different, twice, to people who wrote it down and did not say it out loud. This felt like the same shape, wearing different clothes. Three specialists. Three reasonable opinions. No one, including him, actually deciding anything. And a patient upstairs whose breathing was getting more expensive by the hour.

"I'm going to call all three of them," Elias said.

Maya looked up.

"At the same time. On one line. I want us all talking together, not passing notes back and forth through a chart." He paused. "And I'm going to ask each of them directly what they think the biggest immediate risk is. Not what they recommend in isolation."

The call took twenty minutes to arrange. Pulmonary, cardiology, and Dr. Evans, all three on the line together, Elias on speaker in the workroom, Maya beside him.

"I want to make sure we're solving the same problem," Elias said, once all three were on. "Right now, each of you is managing your own risk. His oxygen requirement has gone from four liters to six since this morning, his gas is worse, and respiratory therapy is asking about high-flow. I need to know which risk is the most immediate for this patient today, so we can choose which danger we're managing first."

There was a brief silence. Then the conversation, for the first time that day, began to move.

Pulmonary spoke first. "His oxygenation is the most acute threat. On that trajectory, he needs intubation within hours, not days."

Cardiology considered this. "If that's the timeline, a small, closely monitored diuresis is more defensible than I initially framed it. I was thinking in terms of days. I can support careful diuresis with pressure checks."

Dr. Evans was quiet. When she spoke, her voice was measured.

"I hear the timeline," she said. "I want to be honest with you about mine. His creatinine has risen twice in forty-eight hours. Diurese him, even carefully, and there is a real chance you convert a struggling kidney into a failing one. Then you are managing respiratory failure and renal failure in the same patient, and dialysis in someone with his blood pressure is not a small thing." She paused. "I understand why you're leaning this way. I can't endorse it. If you do it, do it knowing that my recommendation was to wait."

The line was silent. Two of three was not the clean consensus the phone call had seemed, minutes earlier, to be building toward.

Elias looked at Maya. Then at the phone.

"Then here's the decision," he said. "Low-dose diuresis, starting now. Renal function every four hours. If his creatinine moves more than we can defend, we stop and reassess with all three of you back on the line. If his oxygenation hasn't improved in six hours, we escalate. Dr. Evans, I heard you, and I'm writing your recommendation into my note exactly as you gave it. This is my decision, not a committee's. If it goes wrong, it goes wrong on my order."

"That's all I ask," Evans said. "Check the labs. Call me at the first bump, not the second."

The room, even over the phone, seemed to loosen. A plan, finally, that belonged to someone.

The diuresis worked. Not cleanly — the creatinine rose overnight, enough that Elias was on the phone with Evans at two in the morning, walking through the numbers, adjusting the dose, defending the decision he had made out loud twelve hours earlier. But the oxygen requirement fell. Six liters became four, then two. Intubation, which had felt that morning like an inevitability arriving on its own schedule, was avoided entirely. The kidney recovered over the following days, slowly, the way Evans had predicted it might if the diuresis was gentle and somebody was watching. The patient left the unit five days later, weaker than he had been, breathing on his own, walking with assistance down the hallway on his way to a step-down unit.

That evening, Lighthouse found Elias and Maya in the workroom. He had heard about the call.

"Three consultants on one line, asked to name the most immediate risk," he said. He watched Elias. "That is not how most residents handle three competing opinions."

"It didn't end the way I expected," Elias said. "I thought if I got them talking, they'd agree. Two of them did. Evans didn't, and she was right not to — his creatinine went up, exactly the way she said it might."

"And yet you proceeded."

"Somebody had to. Waiting was also a decision. It just would have been one nobody signed."

Lighthouse weighed it. "Diffusion of responsibility does not require bad specialists," he said. "It requires only good specialists, each managing their own narrow risk, with no one managing the whole patient. What you did on that call was not getting them to agree. Agreement is pleasant when it happens. What you did was take the decision out of the seams between their notes and put your name on it, where Dr. Evans could hold you to it." He paused. "She called you at two in the morning."

"I called her."

"Better still," Lighthouse said. "Owning a decision is not a single moment. It is answering for it afterward, at inconvenient hours, to the person who told you not to make it."

Maya spoke. "I asked the question. What are we doing. I didn't have the next step myself."

"You didn't need to," Lighthouse said. "The question matters even when you are not the one who answers it. Someone has to ask it before someone else can act on it." He looked between them. "The two of you are starting to do this without me in the room."

It was not quite praise. It was something closer to an observation, offered plainly, the way Lighthouse offered most things that mattered.

That night, Elias wrote in his notebook.

Three good opinions are not the same as one good plan.
Someone has to own the decision, out loud, on the record
— especially when the smartest person on the line disagrees.
Owning it includes the two a.m. phone call
when her prediction starts coming true.

Maya, in her own notebook, wrote something shorter.

Asking "what are we doing"
is not the same as answering it.
But it is sometimes the only thing
that makes someone else finally answer.

Clinical Reflection

Diffusion of responsibility rarely involves incompetence — more often several skilled specialists, each reasoning soundly within their own domain, each optimizing their own slice of the risk. The danger lives in the seams, where no one has been asked to hold the whole patient. The sum of individually minimized risks is not a plan; it is a stalemate with a deteriorating patient inside it. The reflex is to manufacture consensus, so the decision belongs to the group and its consequences to no one. But some decisions must be made over a standing objection — made legitimate not by confidence but by transparency: name the dissent, and answer for it personally. Gather every opinion, then let one person state the plan and own it aloud. A patient cared for by everyone in general is cared for by no one in particular.

PART II — CHAPTER 11

What Experience Forgets

The Patient Nobody Would Examine

The most damaging closure
is not the one that names the wrong diagnosis.
It is the one that never completes the examination.
And calls that medicine.

He came back by ambulance. That was the difference between this visit and the last two. He could no longer drive himself. Could no longer walk to a waiting room, sit in a plastic chair, and wait his turn like anyone else. He arrived on a stretcher.

Forty-two years old. Over four hundred pounds. Blood pressure eighty systolic. Heart rate one twenty-two. Temperature one-oh-four point one. Septic, source unknown.

The ER team moved efficiently. Fluids wide open. Blood cultures drawn. Broad-spectrum antibiotics hung within twenty minutes. Good medicine. Fast medicine. Medicine practiced on the parts of the patient that were accessible.

Maya Chen was four weeks into her second emergency medicine rotation, ten months into her intern year and beginning to show — the pregnancy that would take her off the service in only a few months, though she was still working full shifts and meant to until the last of them" She had been assigned to this patient by the supervising resident with the economy of a busy ER night. "Get a history," the resident said. "I'll be back."

Maya pulled up a chair. She sat with him. He was uncomfortable, breathing fast, pain present but hard to localize.

"Where does it hurt," she asked.

He shifted. "Down there," he said. Vague. Embarrassed. The economy of a man describing something in a place he had not been able to examine himself for longer than he wanted to admit.

Maya wrote it down. Pain — perineal/groin region. Difficult to localize. Then she looked at the chart. Two prior encounters. Eight days ago. Five days ago. She read the notes carefully.

The first note documented his weight in the first three lines. The physical examination section read four words. Exam limited by patient size. The second note had no examination documented at all.

Maya read both notes twice. She had not yet accumulated the habits that allow experienced clinicians to accept what cannot be done as a substitute for what must be. She found the resident.

"I think we need a CT," she said.

The resident looked up from another chart. "We're already treating empirically. Broad coverage. Fluids running."

"He has perineal pain," Maya said. "Two prior visits. No examination documented either time."

The resident paused. Looked at her. Then picked up the phone.

The radiology technician picked up on the third ring.

"He's four hundred and twelve pounds," the resident said. "We need an abdomen and pelvis."

A pause on the other end. "Our table limit is three-fifty."

"I understand. But he's septic without a source and we can't examine him adequately."

"I understand that. But if he exceeds the weight limit and something happens on the table —"

"Something is already happening," the resident said.

Another pause. Longer. Maya stood beside the resident. She had followed him to the phone. She did not look away. The resident glanced at her. Something in her expression. Not pressure. Not urgency in the ordinary sense. Certainty. The certainty of someone who does not yet know that some battles are not worth fighting and is therefore still willing to fight them.

Dr. Elara Holt was the attending on call. She had been called for the admission and had come down to the ER. Maya filled her in on the patient's story.

Elara took the phone. "We need this scan," she said. "I'll take responsibility."

They found a way. A different scanner. A different table. A different room down the hall that could barely accommodate him. It took forty minutes to arrange. Maya stayed with the patient while they waited. She did not have a diagnosis. She had never seen Fournier's gangrene. Had barely heard the term. She had only a patient with perineal pain, two prior visits where nobody had looked, and a certainty she could not yet name that the source of his sepsis was in the place nobody had examined.

The scan took eleven minutes. The images came up on the screen at the nursing station at eleven forty-seven.

Dr. Holt and Maya stood at the scanner workstation. They turned to the images. Gas tracking through the perineal fascia. Extensive. Bilateral. The unmistakable signature of an infection that had been present, and advancing, for longer than anyone wanted to calculate.

Elara did not answer right away. The resident was beside her, and the surgical resident who had been paged. Maya stood at the edge of the group. The room was quiet — not the quiet of confusion, the quiet of recognition. Elara let it hold. One breath. Two. Then she turned to the resident.

"He needs the OR," she said. "Tonight."

The surgery resident was already reaching for his phone to call his attending. The room moved.

The surgery lasted four hours. The infection had tracked further than the scan suggested. He went to the ICU afterward. Intubated, on two pressors, with the fragility of a man whose body had been fighting something for eight days without help. He was in the ICU for six weeks.

He survived.

Three days later, Elara sat in the workroom. Late, after rounds, the building quieter than it had been. She read through the three prior encounters. The first ER note. Exam limited by patient size. The office note. No examination documented. The return visit notes before the scan. Labs. Cultures. Antibiotics. No perineal examination.

She sat with the notes for a long time. She did not write anything. She did not call a conference. Did not draft a protocol. Did not compose the teaching email that part of her felt the situation required. She sat with the discomfort — the particular discomfort of understanding that a man had been seen three times, by careful clinicians, in good institutions, and had nearly died not because the diagnosis was obscure but because the examination was never completed, and nobody had named that as the problem it was.

He had been heavy. Difficult. Inconvenient in the way of patients whose bodies make the work of medicine harder than it is supposed to be. And somewhere in the accumulated weight of three encounters, that knowledge had done something quiet and corrosive to the urgency everyone felt about finding his answer.

She did not say this to anyone. She held it, the way a new attending would hold things that are too large for a hallway conversation and too important to reduce to a case conference slide.

A week later she found Maya writing notes at the nursing station. She sat down beside her.

"The scan," Elara said.

Maya looked up.

"You pushed for it."

Maya nodded. "Thank you for trusting me. I didn't know what I was looking for. I just knew we hadn't looked."

Elara was quiet. "That was enough," she said.

Maya looked at her. "He had been seen twice before," she said carefully. "And nobody examined him." It was not quite a question.

Elara held the silence. "No," she said. "They didn't."

She did not elaborate. She did not assign blame, did not offer explanation, did not reach for the comfortable absolution of systemic complexity or institutional limitation or the genuine difficulty of examining a four-hundred-pound patient in a busy emergency department at two in the morning. She simply confirmed what Maya already knew. And let her sit with it.

That night, Maya wrote in her notebook.

We could not examine him.
That was not the end of the obligation.
It was the beginning of it.
He almost didn't make it.
Because he was heavy.
And we let that matter more than it should have.

She closed the notebook. She did not sleep well. She did not think she was supposed to.

Clinical Reflection

Experience is supposed to prevent diagnostic error. In its most advanced form it produces one — not through ignorance but through the confidence of a clinician who has seen enough to stop looking where the answer still lives. The exam is declared impossible, the workup proceeds on whatever remains accessible, and the incompleteness is accepted as though incomplete were the same as sufficient. The documentation is where this hides in plain sight. "Exam limited by patient size" is not a conclusion; it is an unfinished sentence. The complete one is: exam limited — therefore the following alternative was pursued. Any barrier that ends the sentence rather than redirecting it has turned a logistical problem into a diagnostic verdict. The instinct that defeats this erodes with exactly the experience meant to confer it. Guard it accordingly.

PART II — CHAPTER 12

The Discipline of Pause

What Maya Learns to Hold

The pause is not delay. It is permission.
The first answer belongs to the room.
The truth may need someone to stay.

It was the last week of June. Maya Chen was days from the end of her intern year, and weeks away from something larger — the leave that would take her out of the hospital for the first extended time since she had started, the pregnancy now unmistakable, the countdown to it running quietly underneath every shift. She had reached the point where the work had become familiar enough to trust and not yet so familiar that she had stopped watching.

A new intern in orientation had joined the team that week, rotating through before the real weight of internship arrived for him in just a few days. His name was Noah. Quiet. Watchful. The alertness of someone trying to absorb everything at once, uncertain yet which details would turn out to matter. He shadowed them closely that week, saying little, noticing more than he let on.

The patient was a sixty-three-year-old woman. Fatigue. Weight loss. Intermittent fevers, low-grade, the kind that come and go without ever fully resolving. The physical exam was unremarkable, except for her teeth — several in poor repair, one recently extracted. No one took note of that finding. The workup was incomplete. Labs suggestive, not definitive. Blood cultures showed only a skin contaminant. Imaging ambiguous. The story unfinished, in the way that some stories take longer to tell than a single admission allows for.

On rounds, Elias listened as Maya presented. "Sixty-three-year-old female, fatigue and weight loss, intermittent low-grade fevers. Workup so far unrevealing." She paused. The room waited. Noah watched from the back, absorbing the silence that followed, not yet understanding that the silence itself was doing some of the work.

"I don't know yet," Maya said. The words came out steadier than she expected. "I'd like to gather more before we name anything."

Elias felt something ease in his chest, hearing her say it. He did not speak. He let her plan stand without adding to it — the restraint he had learned, two years earlier, from someone who had once done the same for him.

That afternoon, Maya returned to the room alone, between other tasks, the way she had learned to do across this entire year when something about a case asked for more time than rounds alone could offer it. The patient was resting, her husband having stepped out for coffee.

"How are you feeling," Maya asked, sitting down, not standing the way a quick check would have her stand.

The patient considered the question. "Tired," she said. "Mostly just tired. And there's something I haven't told anyone here."

Maya waited. She did not fill the silence. She had learned, by now, that silence held open was often the only thing that made room for what came next.

"A long time ago," the patient said, "I used drugs. Intravenously. It's been years. I got clean. I built a whole life on the other side of it. I didn't want anyone here to look at me differently because of something that isn't who I am anymore." She studied Maya. "But I think it might matter. For whatever this is."

Maya nodded slowly. "Thank you for telling me," she said. She did not rush to reassure. She did not promise it would not be written down, because she knew, already, that it would need to be — carefully, in a way that served the diagnosis without becoming the entire story of who this woman was.

"I'm not proud of it. I never told my husband."

Maya examined her hands more closely after that, the way she had not thought to before, when the history had not yet given her a reason to look in this direction. Small, dark, linear marks beneath several fingernails. Splinter hemorrhages. Subtle. Easy to miss on a hand that nobody had examined closely, because nobody, until now, had a reason to wonder about her heart valves at all.

Maya sat very still. Endocarditis. Subacute, given the indolent course, the low-grade fevers, the weight loss accumulating slowly rather than announcing itself all at once. A single relapse, six weeks earlier, was enough. It did not require ongoing use. It required only one contaminated exposure, seeding a valve that had been, patiently, declaring itself ever since, in symptoms too vague for anyone to connect to a single afternoon the patient had spent years trying to forget.

She found Elias in the workroom.

"I have something," she said. She told him everything — the disclosure, the timing, the splinter hemorrhages, the picture that was beginning, finally, to cohere.

Elias listened without interrupting. When she finished, he sat with it.

"You went back alone," he said.

"I did."

"And you didn't push when she didn't volunteer it the first time."

"I waited," Maya said. "I think she needed to know I wasn't going anywhere before she said it."

They made one more decision that afternoon, and it was Maya who proposed it. The patient was stable. She had been stable for weeks. Starting broad antibiotics now, before the organism declared itself, risked sterilizing the cultures and leaving them treating a diagnosis they could never confirm.

"Three sets of cultures," Maya said. "Drawn separately, over today and tonight. Antibiotics after the third set. Not before."

It was, in its own way, the harder order to write — the deliberate decision not to treat, for a defined interval, in a patient everyone now suspected was infected. Elias co-signed it without amendment.

An echocardiogram was ordered. It would take two more days for the full picture to confirm itself — vegetations on the mitral valve, all three culture sets growing a viridans streptococcus, consistent with exactly the kind of subacute, slowly accumulating infection that explained every symptom that had refused, until now, to organize itself into anything nameable.

Noah watched all of this from the edges of the team, saying little, though Elias noticed him taking careful notes during the conversation in the workroom — the attentiveness of someone deciding, what kind of physician he wanted to become.

"You didn't say anything today," Elias said to him, near the end of the day.

Noah looked up, slightly startled. "I didn't think I had anything worth adding."

"You will," Elias said.

It was not quite reassurance. It was something closer to a promise, offered the way such things are usually offered — without either person fully understanding yet how true it would turn out to be.

That evening, Lighthouse stopped by briefly, having heard that something had resolved itself on the service that day. He did not ask for the full case. He looked at Maya.

"You said I don't know yet, in front of the whole team," he said.

"I did," Maya said.

"How did it feel."

She considered this honestly. "Uncomfortable. For about a day. Then it felt like the only honest thing I could have said."

Lighthouse nodded. "That discomfort," he said, "is the entire discipline. Not the absence of it. The willingness to hold it anyway, long enough for the truth to have room to arrive."

He looked between Maya and Elias. "This is the last week of June," he said. It was not really a question.

"I know," Elias said.

"A new year begins on Tuesday," Lighthouse said. He watched Noah, still standing quietly near the door, and at Maya. "And a new chapter for others."

That night, Maya opened her notebook for what she understood, without being told, was the last entry of her intern year. She had filled most of it. Coherence. Compression. Dissonance. Authority. Groupthink. Ease. Deviance. Protocol. Disengagement. Diffusion. Closure. And now, on the final page, she wrote the lesson that seemed to hold all the others together.

She trusted me with something she had been afraid to say.
I held still long enough to let her say it.
That stillness was not weakness.
It was the only thing that worked.

She closed the notebook. She did not open a new one yet.

Elias, in his own notebook, wrote a shorter line, beneath everything he had written across two full years now.

I taught her to say I don't know yet.
She taught me that saying it well
is a medicine in itself.

He thought of Noah, quiet by the door, a few days from his own July first, a few years from understanding what this week had been. He closed the notebook. Outside, somewhere, new badges were already waiting, for a new group of interns crossing over that threshold.

Clinical Reflection

The discipline of pause doesn't announce itself as a technique. It feels like discomfort — the vulnerability of saying I don't know yet in front of a team expecting something decisive. Every incentive in training runs the other way: presentations reward conclusions, rounds reward plans, and a differential that ends in honest uncertainty can sound like failure when it is often the only accurate summary of the evidence. This is the discipline that holds all the others together. Nearly every failure in this book has the same moment at its root: the mind closing before the evidence did, because something made stopping feel safe — a fluent answer, a senior voice, a familiar pattern, a running checklist, an agreeing room. Each of those is a different door, and they all close the same way. The pause is the one habit that keeps every one of them open a moment longer: not indecision, not delay for its own sake, but the trained capacity to stay in the question after every instinct says to leave it. Learn this, and you need not memorize the rest. Everything else in these pages is only a specific case of it.

The Anatomy of Error

The Traps, Named and Gathered

Every trap in this book is a way of thinking that stopped too soon. Here each one is named, with the single question or discipline that reopens it — meant to be carried, not memorized. The page you return to when a case feels finished and something still nags.

Part I — The Seduction of the First Answer

1. Premature Closure. Once the first answer fits, ask what it does not explain. If the answer is something, let it reopen the case.
2. Anchoring Bias. Before the exam begins, ask what would make this not the diagnosis already attached to the patient — then look as if you had never seen the chart.
3. Confirmation Bias. When a patient corrects their own complaint, stop. That moment is not a detail; it is the diagnosis asking to be reconsidered.
4. Search Satisfaction. When a patient stays sicker than the answer accounts for, the gap is the diagnosis, still waiting. Ask when the finding first appeared.
5. Framing Effect. The most dangerous labels are not diagnoses at all. Close the chart, pull up a chair, and ask the one question the label made unnecessary.
6. Availability Bias. The last case you saw is the first one you see again. Before the room fills and the mind follows, ask what would make this not the case you remember most vividly.

7. Representativeness. A famous finding everyone looks for and does not find proves little. Ask what single diagnosis fits everything in the room — not most of it, all of it.
8. Overconfidence. The week you feel sharpest is the week to be most careful. Reopen the chart on the strength of the one detail the answer cannot explain.
9. Diagnosis Momentum. Inheriting a diagnosis is not the same as earning it. Every handoff is a chance to reset; ask what the momentum never stopped to ask.
10. Time Pressure. The watching is the treatment. Never let a private room and a quiet order be mistaken for the surveillance they remove.
11. Outcome Bias. Improvement tells you the first diagnosis was right, not that the story is finished. Ask what the new findings share.
12. Hindsight Bias. Judge every decision by what was known when it was made. Then find the question that was missing, and make it yours.

Part II — The Erosion of Thinking

13. Narrative Coherence. Trust a story less because it explains everything. Test it with one question it was never asked to answer.
14. Narrative Compression. When a case will not come together, ask the same question a second time — and stay long enough to hear the answer that does not come in the first thirty seconds.
15. Cognitive Dissonance. When a note begins describing the historian instead of the history, the patient has been reclassified. Ask whether the inconsistency belongs to the patient or the disease.
16. Authority Bias. The discomfort of disagreement is not evidence that you are wrong. Ask the question aloud, where someone with the standing to be wrong must answer it.
17. Groupthink. Consensus never opposed is not a verdict. Before a diagnosis closes, assign one person, aloud, to argue the best case against it.
18. Cognitive Ease. When a story repeats for the third time, give it the workup you would give a first encounter. Mistaking ease for evidence is the danger, not the ease itself.

19. Normalization of Deviance. When an abnormal finding stops feeling alarming, ask what would have to be true for this time to be different. Then check whether it already is.
20. Protocol Fixation. When a patient says this is different, stop and ask what the protocol was never built to ask. Even when every box is checked — especially then.
21. Moral Disengagement. Every admission deserves the first one's workup — not because the patient demands it, but because the disease does not know it is not the first.
22. Diffusion of Responsibility. Gather every opinion, then let one person state the plan and own it aloud. A patient cared for by everyone in general is cared for by no one in particular.
23. The Unfinished Exam. "Exam limited" is not a conclusion; it is a sentence that must end in — therefore this alternative was pursued. A barrier is not a verdict.

The Discipline That Holds the Rest

The Discipline of Pause. The willingness to say I don't know yet, and to keep the door open after every instinct says to close it. Nearly every trap in this book has the same moment at its root: the mind closing before the evidence did. This is the one habit that answers them all.

Part III

What We Leave Behind

There is a moment in every training program when the direction of attention reverses.

The intern who spent two years watching becomes the chief resident who is watched. The questions that once arrived from someone standing at the back of the room now arrive from someone standing at the front of it. The transition is administrative on paper. It is something else entirely in practice.

Elias Ward is chief resident now. He runs morning report. He takes the three a.m. calls from interns who are not yet sure what they are looking at. He stands in the hallway after difficult cases and says the things that need to be said to people who are not yet ready to say them to themselves. He does this the way he was taught — which is to say, imperfectly, with the habits that formed in him during two years of watching someone else do it, carrying forward the parts he understood and, without realizing it, the parts he didn't.

Maya Chen will return from three months away. She is quieter in some ways. More certain in others. The patience she brought back from a different kind of learning shows up in the rooms she enters and in the questions she asks before anyone else has thought to ask them.

Noah Reyes is the new intern. He is watching everything. He does not yet know what he is absorbing.

And Lighthouse is still here. But he is spending more time in doorways than in rooms. Watching what has taken root. Checking, without announcing that he is checking, whether the habit he spent a career modeling has traveled far enough to survive without him.

That is the question Part III asks.

Not whether the teaching was good. Not whether the cases were instructive. But whether what passed between one person and another — in hallways, at bedsides, in workrooms at three in the morning — was real enough to keep moving after the person who started it has stepped back.

You do not get to know the answer while you are still teaching.

You find out when you stand in the doorway and watch what happens in the room you chose not to enter.

PART III — CHAPTER 1

What Survives the Teacher

Noah's First Night

Every clinician inherits a way of thinking.
Not just from textbooks.
From people.
Sometimes it is the patient
Who is the teacher.

Sunlight cut through the tall windows of Westside Hospital. July first. The day medicine rearranged itself, the way it did every year, on a schedule that did not pause for anyone's readiness.

At the center of the room stood Dr. Elias Ward. Chief resident now.

"For the next year," he said, "you'll rotate through services covering most of what this hospital does. Some of you will work under Dr. Henry Lighthouse."

A few interns shifted, the way interns always shifted at that name, even now — the stories sharpening and softening the way stories do once they no longer belong to anyone who was there.

The door opened. Not Lighthouse. Dr. Elara Holt, staff attending, returning today only as a favor, to help cover an attending shortage on morning report.

"I didn't know you were covering today," Elias said.

"Neither did I, until three days ago," Elara said, smiling. "I heard you were running the show now." She looked at the new interns.

"Good luck. You're about to learn that the answers matter less than you think, and the questions matter more than anyone tells you on the first day."

Among them stood Noah. Quiet. Watchful. Today he was simply one more new badge, tablet in hand, standing in a room that did not yet know his name.

His first call came just after eight that evening. Fifty years old. A bank vice president. Jaundiced, with abnormal liver enzymes and the yellow cast to his skin that made everyone in the room think the same word before anyone said it.

Noah took the history carefully. Melanoma, five years prior. Wide excision. Clean margins. His oncologist had told him, at the five-year mark, that he could consider himself in remission.

The CT, when it came back, showed otherwise. Multiple liver metastases. Innumerable, the radiologist's read said. The melanoma had not gone anywhere. It had simply waited.

Noah delivered this news with Elias beside him — the weight of being the one who has to say the words that change the rest of someone's life in a single sentence.

The patient took it differently than Noah expected. Calm. Almost matter of fact.

"I was a company commander in the Army, a long time ago, Iraq, then Afghanistan," he said, when Noah asked how he was holding up. "I lost men — more than I ever thought I would. I am not afraid of this. I have already seen what it looks like. This is just my turn."

Noah sat with him for a while after Elias left to cover the other ward.

"How do you do that," Noah asked. "Just decide not to be afraid."

The man considered the question. "You don't decide it all at once," he said. "You decide it the first time, when you're young, and someone next to you doesn't make it. After that, it's not really a decision anymore. It's just something you know." He turned to Noah. "You'll learn your own version of that. This work will teach it to you, whether you're ready or not."

Elias found Noah in the workroom near midnight, between admissions.

"How are you doing," he asked.

"I don't know yet," Noah said honestly.

Elias nodded. "That's the right answer," he said. "Tonight, anyway."

That night, in the first entry of a notebook he had only just begun keeping, Noah wrote a few lines.

Some patients teach you
before you've learned anything about how to help them.
I don't know what to do with that yet.
I'm going to keep it anyway.

Clinical Reflection

Most chapters here end with something the clinician should have done differently. This one does not, because nothing was done wrong. A man received devastating news and carried it with a steadiness his intern could not yet imagine — and the intern learned something no case presentation could teach. The lesson is not clinical. It is that the people we are trained to help sometimes have more to teach us about facing what cannot be fixed than we have to offer them in return. That is not a failure of medicine. It is one of its oldest, quietest truths.

PART III — CHAPTER 2

The Wrong Hands

What Elias Would Not Sign Off On

Authority does not make hands steady.
It only makes them harder to stop.
Someone still must be willing to stand in the way.

The patient was Sage. Seventy-one years old. Small. Frail in a way that made her seem, somehow, more vulnerable than her vitals alone suggested — the fragility that makes an experienced nurse glance twice without being able to say exactly why.

The pain had been vague all day. That was, in part, why it took until evening for anyone to feel the concern that finally moved the workup forward. Mid-upper abdomen. Dull. Intermittent. Murphy's sign negative. No rebound. No guarding. A reasonable clinician, reading the exam alone, could have waited until morning.

Noah was the one who pushed for imaging. "Something about her color," he said to Elias, in the hallway, between two other patients. "And she winces when she breathes in deep, even without me pressing anywhere."

"Order the stat CT," Elias said.

The scan showed fluid around the gallbladder, a single large stone, wall thickening. The radiologist's read used the word concerning. Possible gangrenous cholecystitis. A surgical emergency if the read was right. Surgery was called just after midnight.

The senior surgery resident on call arrived nearly forty minutes later. Elias noticed it before anyone said anything. The unsteadiness in his gait, crossing the workroom. The slight delay in his speech. The smell of alcohol, faint but unmistakable, beneath the breath spray he had clearly used in the elevator on his way up.

"Where's the chart," the resident said, his voice carrying the overcorrected steadiness of someone trying very hard to sound entirely normal.

Elias handed him the chart. He watched him scan it, too quickly.

"I'll take her up," the resident said. "Get her consented."

"I don't think that's a good idea," Elias said.

The room went quiet.

"This is my case now," the resident said, straightening, his voice gaining an edge. "Surgery overrules medicine. You don't get a vote here."

"I'm not voting," Elias said, keeping his voice level. "I'm telling you what I'm seeing. You've been drinking. I can smell it. Your speech is slow."

"Are you accusing me of something," the resident said, stepping closer.

"I'm not letting you operate on my patient tonight," Elias said.

"You don't get to make that call. I outrank you. This isn't your specialty."

"It's my patient," Elias said. "Until she's in your operating room, she is my responsibility. And I am telling you, clearly, that you are not fit to take her there."

The resident shoved him. A hand to the chest, hard enough to push Elias back half a step, not hard enough to be anything but what it obviously was — a man losing the argument the only way his judgment, impaired as it was, could still find to fight back.

The room froze. A nurse near the desk had already reached for the phone. Noah did not move; he had no script for this.

Nobody spoke. Elias did not raise his hands. He did not step forward again. He simply stood there, steady, and said nothing, letting the silence do something his words had not yet managed.

Something shifted in the resident's face. The anger began to fold inward, replaced by something that looked, for the first time, like the beginning of understanding — what he had just done, in front of how many witnesses, and what it would mean for the career he had spent a decade building toward.

He stood there a moment longer. Then he reached for his phone. He called his attending. His voice was quiet now, the overcorrected steadiness gone. He explained the case briefly. He did not explain what had happened in the room. He did not need to.

"I can't take this case tonight," he said.

A pause. Then he hung up.

He stood in the doorway, his hand on the frame. He did not look back. Then he was gone — through the doors, into the parking structure, into the night that was already writing the next chapter of his career without his permission.

The attending arrived twelve minutes later. The resident's call had told her only that he couldn't take the case — not why. She came through the doors quickly and stopped.

She read the room in a single pass. The nurse still near the phone. Noah against the wall. Elias standing in the center of it. Steady. Still holding the charge of it. The absent resident, whose absence explained everything.

She did not ask what had happened. She looked at Elias. One look. Brief. The look of a senior clinician who has seen this before, or known someone who has, or understands, in the way people who have spent decades in operating rooms understand, exactly what this night was going to cost the young man who was no longer in it.

She held it. Then she turned to the junior surgery resident, who had arrived quietly behind her.

"Let's go see the patient," she said.

The gallbladder was removed without complication, the gangrenous changes confirmed exactly as the imaging had suggested. The patient did well.

The next morning, Lighthouse called Elias and Noah into a small office near the administrative suite. He did not ask them what had happened. He asked them to tell it to him again, slowly, from the beginning — each of them, separately, the way a careful clinician takes two histories from two witnesses rather than assuming they will match perfectly.

They did not match perfectly. Small details differed — the exact words, the order of them, whether the shove came before or after the line about rank. The substance did not differ at all.

Lighthouse listened without interrupting. When they finished, he was quiet.

"Thank you," he said. "Both of you."

He picked up the phone on the desk. "I need to speak with the Chief of Surgery," he said, to whoever answered. "This morning, if possible. It's about one of his residents."

He studied Elias while he waited to be connected. "You did the right thing last night," he said. "I want you to hear that clearly, before anything else happens today, because what happens next will not always feel like confirmation of that."

That night, Noah wrote in his notebook.

Rank is not the same as correctness.
You must know, before it happens,
that you will say something
even when the person you are saying it to outranks you by years.
Deciding that in the moment is too late.
Decide it now, long before you need it.

Clinical Reflection

Hierarchy in medicine exists for reasons often sound, but it is not infallible, and an impaired clinician does not become safe to operate simply because he outranks the person raising the concern. The people most likely to notice impairment are frequently the least powerful in the room — interns, residents, nurses — who see it first and have the least standing to act. The cost of speaking is real; the cost of silence is measured in patients placed in the wrong hands. The ground to stand on is narrow and specific: not character, not accusation, but observable findings stated plainly, and the one decision that is genuinely yours to make. Decide now — before you are tired, before the room is stacked against you — that patient safety outranks every other kind of rank there is.

PART III — CHAPTER 3

When Criteria Are Not Enough

Before I Go Home

Not every request needs to be explained
before it deserves an answer.
Some things a patient knows
that no chart will ever record.

Mr. Jones had terminal lung cancer. That was not a surprise to anyone, least of all to him. He had been admitted three days earlier for the effects of the latest round of chemotherapy — a round he had pressed for himself, against gentle advice, with the tiny hope he still clung to. The hardest conversation there is to have had already been had, with his family and with the team. He had listened to all of it, agreed with most of it, and still declined the "No Code" designation. Nobody pushed. Some things a man is entitled to hold onto while he decides how to let go.

Noah had seen him that afternoon. Arterial blood gases, drawn carefully from the wrist the way every intern learns during the exhaustion of a long call night. Normal. Oxygenation adequate. No clinical indication for supplemental oxygen at all.

The page came at one in the morning.

"Mr. Jones says he needs oxygen," the nurse said.

Noah walked to the room, already turning over in the tired arithmetic of a brain running on no sleep the fact that he had confirmed, hours earlier, that oxygen was not indicated.

"I know I need oxygen," he said. "Before I go home."

Noah sat down. "Mr. Jones," he said gently, "your oxygen levels are good. You're not going home tomorrow. We'll make all the arrangements before that happens."

"But I need oxygen," Mr. Jones said. "Before I go home."

He said it without urgency. Without argument. The quiet insistence of a man repeating something he was certain of, regardless of whether the person across from him understood why.

Noah reassured him as best he could and left to admit the next patient waiting in the emergency department.

The second page came an hour later. The nurse's voice carried the fatigue of someone managing more than one demanding situation at the same time. Noah explained again that the blood gases did not support it. He was certain he was right. He had the numbers. He went back to his admissions.

The third page came near three.

By then Noah had been awake for over twenty hours. He found Elias in the workroom, reviewing a chart between rounds on two different wards.

"Mr. Jones keeps asking for oxygen," Noah said. "His gases are normal. I don't have a clinical reason to give it."

Elias looked up. He did not ask for the numbers.

"Is he in distress," he said.

"Not really. Just insistent. He says he needs it before he goes home."

Elias was quiet.

"Give him the oxygen," he said.

Noah hesitated. "It's not indicated —"

"He's dying," Elias said. "It won't hurt him. And you've been saying no to a dying man for three hours. Sometimes the kindest thing isn't the thing that fits the criteria. Give him the oxygen, I'll handle the rest."

Noah ordered the oxygen. Two liters, by nasal cannula. A small thing, clinically speaking. He did not think about it again for almost two hours, buried in admissions, the tunnel that a long call night narrows into, where each task exists only in relation to the one before it and the one after.

The code call came at five.

Harvey team, seven east.

Noah ran. By the time he arrived the room was full, the team already moving through compressions, through the practiced choreography of a code in progress. It did not work. The time was called a few minutes later. The nurse explained afterward that Mr. Jones had become acutely short of breath, then collapsed — the way some endings arrive without much warning even when they are, in another sense, not unexpected at all.

Noah stood in the hallway in the stillness that follows a code that does not end the way anyone hoped. He thought of the oxygen. Of the three pages. Of his own certainty, hours earlier, that he was right to withhold something that did not meet criteria. He did not yet know whether any of it had mattered.

That morning, Elias found Noah before he went home.

"Come with me," he said. "I want to talk to his wife."

She was sitting in a small family room, composed — the composure of someone who had had days, not hours, to begin preparing for what had just happened. Elias sat across from her. Noah stood near the door.

"I wanted to tell you what happened overnight," Elias said. He explained it plainly. The pages. The oxygen. The collapse. He did not soften it, and he did not dramatize it.

She listened carefully. When he finished, she was quiet.

"He told me, he knew he was near the end," she said, "that he was ready to go home."

Noah felt something tighten in his chest.

"He was a preacher," she said, looking at them. "For over thirty years. When he said home, he didn't mean the house we've lived in. He meant Heaven. He'd been telling me that for days. That he was going home soon." She paused. "The oxygen — he told me that morning that he needed it before he went home. I think it made it easier. Easier to breathe, at the very end, on his way there."

Noah did not say anything. He did not trust his voice to hold steady if he tried.

Elias nodded slowly. "Thank you for explaining that," he said. "It helps to understand."

Outside in the hallway, Noah finally spoke.

"I almost didn't give it to him. Three times. I almost said no all three times."

"In the end you did, though," Elias said.

"Only because you told me to."

Elias considered this. "That's all right," he said. "You'll learn to trust it yourself eventually. Tonight, you trusted me instead. That's how it starts."

Noah didn't answer. "Do you think he knew," he said. "Not that he was dying. But the breathlessness coming. Do you think he sensed something — and that's why he kept asking."

Elias thought about it honestly. "I don't know," he said, without apology. "There are things patients seem to sense that we can't fully account for. Whether that's what happened here —" He paused. "I don't know."

"Does it matter," Noah asked.

"To medicine," Elias said. "No. To me-" He was quiet. "Yes. A little. It's one of those questions this work leaves you with and doesn't answer."

For a moment he didn't speak. Then he said something he had not said out loud before.

"My mother died my first year of medical school," he said. "A week before she lost consciousness, she was lying in her bed at my home. My father was sitting beside the bed on one side of the room. She was looking at the far wall — not at him, not at me. She said "Daddy." Clearly."

Noah stayed quiet.

"She never called my father Daddy. In forty years of marriage, not once. She used his first name. Always." He paused. "She said it twice, with me in the room. At least once when my wife was there. Different days. Every time she was looking at something none of us could see."

He looked down the hallway. "My father believed for years she was speaking to him. I never told him otherwise."

"Who do you think she was speaking to," Noah asked.

"Her father," Elias said. "She called him Daddy her whole life. He had passed away about six years prior. I believe he was there."

He said it plainly — not a claim that needed defending, just something he had been certain of for a long time.

"You will see things in this work that you cannot make sense of," he said. "Not often. But they come. Hold them. Build your own faith around them, whatever that looks like for you. Medicine does not ask you to explain them." He paused. "But you do not have to let them go."

They stood together in the hallway longer, holding the question between them the way it would need to be held — without resolution, without apology — for the rest of their careers.

That night Noah wrote in his notebook.

I had a reason to say no.
I did not have a reason good enough to keep saying it.
Some requests cannot be explained by the numbers in front of you.
Honor them anyway, when the cost of honoring them is small,
and the cost of refusing might be something
you will never fully understand.

Clinical Reflection

Some judgments appear in no algorithm, because they cannot be standardized without losing the thing that makes them valuable. A dying patient's calm, repeated insistence on something specific is itself a form of information, even when it corresponds to no abnormal value — and it does not always need to be understood to be honored. The calculus is asymmetric: when the cost of honoring the request is negligible and the cost of refusing is unknowable, the numbers are not on the side of refusal; they only feel that way to a mind trained to require an indication for everything. Sometimes the only available response is empathy offered without full comprehension. It often begins the way it began here: someone more experienced saying, let him have it — I'll handle the rest.

PART III — CHAPTER 4

The Question You Inherit

"What Would Make This Not What I Think It Is."

Some habits are taught deliberately.
Others arrive without anyone noticing,
and surface only when you hear yourself
say them to someone else.

The patient was twenty-eight years old. Fever. Cough. Bilateral infiltrates on the chest film — diffuse, patchy, the kind of pattern that fits a familiar story almost too easily.

Noah presented her on rounds, confident, efficient.

"Young woman, fever and cough, bilateral infiltrates. Community-acquired pneumonia, likely atypical organism — Mycoplasma, Chlamydia. Starting azithromycin."

It was a reasonable presentation. The kind that, on a busy morning, draws nods and nothing else.

Elias opened his mouth to agree.

What came out instead surprised him slightly, even as he said it.

"What would make this not pneumonia," he said.

Noah paused. He started to answer, then stopped, turning the question over the way a question asked plainly enough sometimes forces a pause that a more elaborate one would not.

Elias felt something fall into place, hearing himself — a faint, specific recognition he could not immediately locate. He had heard that exact question before. Not asked it. Heard it. A long time ago, in a different workroom, from someone standing where he was standing now.

"No real risk factors for aspiration," Noah said slowly, working through it out loud. "The organisms I'm treating for don't usually cause this degree of bilateral involvement this quickly. And the eosinophil count was elevated on the differential — I didn't flag it. It didn't seem like the main story."

"What's eosinophilia not usually a feature of," Elias said.

"Community-acquired pneumonia." Noah looked up. "You think this isn't infectious."

"I think we should find out what would make it not be," Elias said, "before we commit fully to a story that fits well enough to stop us from checking."

A CT was ordered that afternoon. Peripheral ground-glass opacities — a pattern distinct from the consolidative picture typical infection usually produces. Not infection. Inflammatory. Eosinophilic pneumonia, confirmed shortly after by bronchoalveolar lavage, the eosinophil count unmistakable once someone went looking for it.

Steroids were started. The response, within hours, was dramatic.

That evening Elias sat in the workroom — the same one that had outlasted several years of trainees passing through it. He thought about the question again.

What would make this not.

He could not remember, specifically, the first time he had heard it. He only knew with certainty that he had not invented it.

Noah found him there.

"That question you asked this morning," Noah said. "Where did you learn to ask it that way."

Elias considered this honestly. "I'm not entirely sure," he said. "I think I heard it enough times, early on, that it stopped being something I was taught and became something I just do now."

"From Lighthouse," Noah said. It was not quite a question.

"Probably," Elias said. "I couldn't point you to the exact day. That might be the strangest part of it. The things that change how you think rarely arrive as a single dramatic lesson. They arrive enough that you don't notice you've kept them until you hear yourself handing them to someone else."

Noah was quiet.

"I wrote it down tonight," he said. "In my notebook."

"What did you write," Elias asked.

Noah read it aloud.

What would make this not what I think it is.
Ask it before the story closes.
Someday I will ask this without remembering
where I learned it either.

Clinical Reflection

The question that uncovers a hidden diagnosis is seldom a new idea. It is inherited — not through formal instruction but through repeated exposure to someone who asked it often enough, and naturally enough, that it stopped sounding like a lesson and started sounding like instinct. This is how reasoning propagates through a profession: small, repeated questions modeled by people who may not remember teaching them and absorbed by trainees who may not remember learning them, until the question arrives unbidden, exactly when it is needed. The most valuable sentence in this book may be the simplest: what would make this not what I currently believe it to be. Ask it, and keep asking, until someone standing behind you starts asking it too.

PART III — CHAPTER 5

Borrowed Confidence

Often Wrong, Never in Doubt

Confidence can be taught.
Judgment cannot be borrowed the same way.
One travels easily from teacher to student.
The other must be earned the hard way, usually once.

Elias had a way of speaking to frightened patients that Noah had come to admire. Steady. Direct. Never rushed. Even delivering difficult news, Elias rarely sounded uncertain — the calm authority that seemed to quiet a room simply by entering it. Noah had been watching that calm for months, absorbing it the way trainees absorb almost everything, without fully realizing how much of it he was taking in.

The patient was sixty-six years old. A CT ordered for vague abdominal pain showed a mass-like density in the sigmoid colon, irregular borders — the kind of appearance that worried the radiologist enough to use the word concerning twice in one report. Noah reviewed the images himself, carefully, the way he had been taught. The pattern looked to him unmistakably like malignancy.

He sat with her that afternoon. Elias was on a different floor, covering another admission, trusting Noah by now to handle a difficult conversation largely on his own.

"I want to talk to you honestly about what the scan shows," Noah said.

He heard, somewhere underneath his own words, a borrowed steadiness — the tone he had watched Elias use in rooms exactly like this one, many times before.

"This appears to be colon cancer," Noah said. He said it clearly. Steadily. The way Elias would have said it.

The patient's face changed. Fear taking hold at once — the fear that arrives the instant a feared word is finally spoken aloud by someone in a white coat.

"Are you certain," she asked quietly.

"The imaging is very suggestive," Noah said. "We'll need a biopsy to confirm, but I want you to understand what we're likely dealing with."

He believed, saying it, that the calm in his voice was a kindness. A way of giving her something solid to hold onto.

Surgery was scheduled for the following week, the mass requiring resection regardless of final pathology given the degree of obstruction it was beginning to cause. Noah visited her the morning before, still carrying the same certainty he had delivered a week earlier. She held his hand briefly.

"Thank you for being so honest with me," she said. "I've had time to prepare, because of how clearly you explained it."

Noah nodded. Something tightened slightly in his chest that he did not yet have a name for.

The surgery went well. The mass was resected completely. The pathology came back two days later.

Diverticulitis. Severe, with a contained perforation and a small abscess — the inflammatory mass effect mimicking malignancy closely enough to explain the radiologist's concern, closely enough to explain Noah's own certainty, entirely, without a single cancer cell anywhere in the specimen.

Noah read the report several times. He felt, reading it, not relief exactly, though relief was somewhere underneath everything else. He felt foolish. He thought of the conversation a week earlier. This appears to be colon cancer. Said so clearly. So certainly. To a woman who had thanked him sincerely for his honesty, when what he had offered her was confidence wearing the costume of certainty, in a situation that had called for neither.

He found Elias in the workroom.

"I told her it was cancer," Noah said. "Before the biopsy. Before surgery. I told her clearly, like I was certain."

Elias looked up. "What did the pathology show."

"Diverticulitis. An abscess. No malignancy at all." Noah sat down heavily. "I sounded so sure. I don't even know where that came from. I just heard myself say it the way you would have said it."

Elias was slow to answer. "I think I know exactly where that came from," he said. "I learned, a long time ago, from a mentor I respected enormously, that patients trust certainty. He used to say it almost like a motto — often wrong, never in doubt. He meant it as advice about bedside manner. I think I absorbed it as something closer to a method."

"Did you ever do what I just did," Noah asked.

"Once that I remember clearly," Elias said. "A chest CT with a mass-like density in the right upper lobe. I told a patient with complete confidence that I believed it was lung cancer. Surgery showed an inflammatory pseudotumor. Organizing pneumonia, walled off. No cancer. I felt exactly the way you're describing right now."

Noah absorbed this. "Why didn't you ever tell me that."

"Because I didn't realize, until just now, that I had taught you the part of that lesson I was proud of," Elias said, "and left out the part that actually mattered." He looked at Noah. "Confidence is useful. Patients do better, in many situations, with a clinician who can speak clearly and calmly. But confidence is not the same thing as certainty, and you cannot borrow someone else's tone without also borrowing their judgment. I had years of cases behind my own certainty by the time you started watching me. You were copying the sound of it without the years underneath it yet. That was my error to catch, not yours. I should have told you — the calm voice isn't free. It has to be earned, case by case, the same way everything else that matters has to be earned."

That night Noah wrote in his notebook.

I will say "the imaging is concerning"
before I say "this is cancer," until the proof is in my hand.
Borrow the calm.
Earn the certainty separately.

Clinical Reflection

The imaging was read correctly and the suspicion was reasonable; the error was not in the thinking but in the certainty attached to the speaking — borrowed from a mentor's bedside manner without the discrimination that mentor had earned about when such certainty is warranted. Trainees absorb not only their teachers' reasoning but their tone and confidence, which are far easier to copy than the pattern recognition that justifies them. The antidote is not less confidence — patients deserve clarity. It is precision about what the confidence is attached to. Certainty is a currency, and the rule for spending it is simple: attach it to the finding, never to the forecast — to what is in hand, not to what the next test is expected to show. Borrow the calm. Earn the certainty separately, one case at a time.

PART III — CHAPTER 6

The Limits of the Method

When the Disease Asks the Question

Ask one more question.
Widen the lens.
This book has said it in nearly every chapter.
This chapter is about what happens when there isn't time.

The patient was fifty-eight years old. He had spent the afternoon at the state fair, he told Noah, eating his way through it the way a person does once a year, without much thought for consequence. Two Polish sausages, heavy with onions and peppers, sat uneasily somewhere behind his sternum now.

"Chest pain," he said, almost apologetically — the tone of a man who suspects he has brought this on himself. "Feels like reflux, mostly. I've had it before. Just worse this time."

Noah took the history carefully. A known history of GERD. Burning discomfort. Significant belching, which the patient offered up as evidence for his own theory.

"It's the sausages," he said. "I know it is."

The story fit reflux reasonably well. But something about the presentation — the belching itself, the location, the way the patient kept one hand pressed against the center of his chest — kept Noah from closing the question entirely.

"Has the pain moved anywhere," he asked. "Your arm, your jaw, your back."

"Maybe my jaw a little," the patient said. "But that could be anything."

The EKG came back nondiagnostic. No clear ST elevation. Subtle changes in the inferior leads — nothing definitively abnormal, the ambiguity that makes early inferior ischemia one of the more difficult presentations to catch on a single static tracing.

Noah was still working through it, still holding the question open the way he had been taught, when the monitor began to alarm.

Ventricular tachycardia.

The patient's eyes widened. Then he was unresponsive.

Noah called the code. Started chest compressions. There was no time now for one more question. No time to widen anything. There was only the rhythm on the monitor, the pads being placed, the focused narrowing that an emergency demands — where the careful, expansive thinking this entire book has taught simply has no room to operate.

Elias arrived within a minute, just as the nurse was discharging the defibrillator. The shock restored a perfusing rhythm. The patient, dazed and breathing again, was moved emergently toward the cath lab. The working diagnosis was no longer a question of differential possibilities weighed carefully against each other. It was simply: get him to the table.

The catheterization confirmed it. An acute inferior wall myocardial infarction — the right coronary artery occluded near its origin, opened within the hour. The vagal stimulation from the inferior ischemia had explained the belching that seemed, all afternoon, like such convincing evidence for indigestion.

It had never been the sausages.

Noah stood outside the cath lab afterward in the stillness that follows an emergency that moved faster than thought could. Elias found him there.

"You were still taking his history when he went into VT," Elias said.

"I was," Noah said. "I hadn't finished. I was still trying to figure out what would make this not reflux, and then there wasn't time to finish asking."

Lighthouse arrived a short while later, having heard about the code. He watched them.

"You did everything right," he said to Noah, "and the disease still got there first."

Noah looked at him. "I thought the whole point of this work was learning to ask one more question. Before the moment closes."

"It is," Lighthouse said. "Most of the time, you get to ask it. Sometimes the disease asks it for you, and the answer arrives as a rhythm on a monitor instead of a word in a history."

He paused.

"The method does not fail when that happens. It simply runs out of time to finish. Your job in that moment is not to keep asking. It is to recognize that the question has already been answered — urgently, by the patient's own body — and to act on what it is telling you."

"How do you know the difference," Noah asked. "Between a moment that needs more questions and a moment that needs you to stop asking and move."

Lighthouse considered this. "You don't always know in advance," he said. "That is the hardest truth I know. Sometimes you find out the moment required action, not inquiry, only because the monitor tells you so — in the middle of a sentence you didn't get to finish." He turned to Noah. "That is not a failure of the method. It is the method's honest limit. Knowing that limit exists, and not freezing when you meet it, is a skill in itself — separate from the one I have spent so many years teaching."

The patient survived. He recovered well, the right coronary artery patent and flowing by the time he left the hospital a week later. He continued, for years afterward, to tell anyone who asked that it had been the Polish sausages that nearly killed him. Nobody ever fully managed to talk him out of it.

That night Noah wrote in his notebook.

I was still asking the question when the disease answered it for me.
The method did not fail. It simply ran out of road before I did.
I must learn to recognize when the road has ended
and move without finishing the sentence.

Clinical Reflection

Most of this book teaches the pause — one more question, a wider differential, resistance to early closure. This is its limit. Some conditions move faster than any history can be taken; a lethal process in a common costume can declare itself before the clarifying questions are finished. That is not the method failing — it is the method meeting a circumstance it was never built to outrun. The answer is not more questions asked faster. It is recognizing, without hesitation, that the moment for questions has passed and the body has already answered. Widen the lens when you have time. Narrow it instantly, without apology, when you do not.

PART III — CHAPTER 7

What the Junior Sees First

The Pattern Across the Rooms

Hierarchy organizes attention.
It also limits it.
The person without a service,
without a chart already opened,
without a diagnosis already forming
— sometimes sees the whole
before anyone else has finished looking at the parts.

Maya returned on a Tuesday. Three months after her daughter was born, earlier than she'd originally planned — the pull of being a mother meeting the pull of wanting to use her mind again for something she had spent so many years training it to do.

She came back quieter in some ways. More certain in others. Elias noticed it immediately, something in how she moved through a room, the deliberate calm of someone who had spent three months learning patience of a different kind entirely.

She picked up two patients that first morning — one her own, the second while covering for a colleague on leave. Both had been admitted within the past three days, from different services to different floors. She read their charts carefully before she saw the patients themselves. Then she went to see them, one after the other, sitting down each time, asking the questions she had been taught to ask, and then the ones beyond those.

The first patient was sixty-one years old. A woman admitted with acute renal failure, her creatinine rising steadily despite aggressive hydration, no cause identified yet. Maya sat with her for nearly thirty minutes.

"Tell me about your home," she said, at some point toward the end — the kind of question that sounds like small talk and sometimes isn't.

"Recently I've been splitting time at my mother's house," the woman said. "She's terminal. We've been taking turns sitting with her. My sisters and me — four of us, though we don't all get along. Money things. Old things. But someone must be there, so we rotate. A week at a time."

The second patient was fifty-eight years old. Another woman admitted two days earlier with nausea, vomiting, and acute renal failure that had not responded to standard treatment. Maya sat down beside her the way she had sat with the first, and near the end of the history she asked the same question she had asked one floor below.

"Tell me about your home."

"Lately, I've been spending a lot of time at my mother's house," the woman said. "She's dying. My sisters and I take care of her. One week at a time."

Maya stopped. She sat very still.

"How many sisters," she asked.

"Four of us, all together."

Two women. Different last names. Different services, different floors, charts that had never been in the same room together — nothing in either record connecting them to the other. Both with acute renal failure of unclear cause. Both rotating, a week at a time, through the same dying mother's house. The link had not been visible anywhere in the hospital's paperwork. It had surfaced only because the same question had been asked in two rooms by the same person on the same day.

"Is one of your sisters here in the hospital right now," Maya asked.

The woman looked surprised. "Upstairs," she said. "We figured we caught the same bug. Something going around."

Maya found Noah in the workroom. "I need you to help me pull something together," she said. She explained what she had. Noah listened, then began searching — not within either chart, but across the record, looking for anything that touched the same family. He found it within minutes. An emergency department visit, three weeks earlier: the older sister of the two, seen for vomiting and abdominal cramping, given fluids, diagnosed with gastroenteritis, and discharged the same evening. The visit had resolved into nothing. Nobody had connected it to anything, because at the time there had been nothing to connect it to.

"Three episodes," Noah said. "Two sisters. All in the last month. All starting after the caregiving rotation began."

"Could this be infectious. Environmental. The water supply. What do you know about toxins that cause renal failure," Maya said.

Noah thought. "With the GI symptoms first, and then the kidneys — heavy metals," he said slowly. "Lead. Mercury." He paused. "Arsenic."

Maya ordered urine arsenic levels on both patients before she spoke to anyone else. Then she sat down and thought carefully about the weight of what she was suggesting, and what it would mean if she were right.

The levels came back that afternoon. Markedly elevated. Both sisters.

She went to Elias and laid it out plainly, without preamble, without hedging.

"Four sisters. Two of them are upstairs with acute renal failure and confirmed arsenic toxicity. I talked with the third sister. She's a travel nurse, away on a three-month contract — she hasn't taken a rotation since it started — and she's completely well. The fourth we know less about. The youngest. They don't live together. They don't ordinarily eat together. The mother they are caring for is terminal. I am not sure why or if that connects as well. The only place the two in renal failure have shared is their mother's kitchen, and the only food they share is what's left in that refrigerator when each one arrives for her week. The one who is out of town and did not eat at their mother's house is fine. The exposures are too consistent to be a coincidence." She paused. "Could someone be putting arsenic in the food."

The room went still.

Elias called Lighthouse. Lighthouse, after reviewing everything, made two calls simultaneously: the hospital's legal team, and the police.

Officers went to the house that evening. The youngest sister was there, along with her husband. In the mother's refrigerator they found prepared food — casseroles, soups, containers labeled in careful handwriting, left for whichever sister arrived next for her shift. Laced with arsenic. In amounts calculated to sicken slowly rather than kill at once.

The handwriting belonged to the youngest sister. She had been bringing the food for weeks — a kindness, she had called it, so that whoever was sitting with their mother would not have to cook. She took her own rotations like the others. She had simply never eaten from the containers. Her husband had helped her prepare them. The mother's estate was considerable and had been contested among the sisters for years; the husband's gambling had left the two of them in debts he had concealed until concealment stopped being possible. With her sisters too sick to take their rotations — or worse — the care of their mother, and everything that followed from it, narrowed toward her.

The out-of-town sister flew back the next morning. Her account confirmed what the toxicology had already shown: the food preparation had begun the same week the symptoms had. She had missed all of it by the accident of a contract three states away. Then they tested the mother. High arsenic levels as well. The youngest sister and her husband were arrested that night.

Chelation therapy was started on both patients. The road was uncertain for days — the older sister's kidneys had taken the worst of it — but both recovered. Their mother, terminally ill from cancer, died shortly after the discovery. The arsenic speeding up a process that was not happening fast enough for two people desperate enough to do the unthinkable.

Maya sat in the workroom long after the police had gone. Noah found her there.

"You caught it," he said.

"I asked where she lived," Maya said. "And then I recognized the same pattern in the second room. That was all it was."

"That was enough," Noah said.

"I keep thinking," Maya said, "that if I had only seen one of them, I wouldn't have seen anything. The pattern was only visible because I happened to cover both admissions on the same day and asked the same question in both rooms. If they'd stayed on separate services, with separate residents, nobody would have put it together. The ED didn't, three weeks ago. There was no reason to."

Elias came in and sat across from both. "I want to say something to both of you," he said. He looked at Maya first. "You asked a question about home. It was not in any protocol. It was not prompted by any finding. You asked it because you have learned that the story a patient tells you has more rooms in it than the one you're standing in." He studied Noah. "And you looked across the record instead of within it. You found an ED visit that had already closed, and you understood it wasn't closed at all. That is not something most interns think to do."

Lighthouse appeared in the doorway later that evening. He looked at Maya. "You came back after three months from a different kind of work. You are a better clinician today than the one who left. Whatever you learned about sitting still and listening past the obvious answer — you brought it back with you." He watched Noah. "And you looked where nobody else was positioned to look. That is not luck. That is what happens when the right habits meet the right moment."

He left without another word.

That night Maya wrote in her notebook — the same one she had carried through her entire intern year, resumed now with a new section that began with her daughter's birth date at the top of a fresh page.

I asked where she lived. That was all.
The pattern was waiting for someone to cross from one chart to the next.
Hierarchy didn't catch it. Geography did.
A question about home — nothing to do with medicine, everything to do with it.

Noah, in his own notebook, wrote one line.

Look across the rooms, not just into them.

Clinical Reflection

This diagnosis was not reached by knowing more medicine than anyone else in the building. It was reached by looking across a boundary the building is organized to keep people from crossing. Hierarchy focuses care by narrowing it — to this patient, this service, this chart — and that is usually a strength. But some patterns live only in the space between two charts, visible only when one person carries the same question from one room into another. And one habit deserves naming on its own: when something in the environment is making people ill, the person who should be sick and is not is often the more useful subject — a natural experiment the situation has already run for you. Don't only ask who is affected. Ask who ought to be and isn't, and find the one thing they didn't share.

PART III — CHAPTER 8

The Cost of Being Right

What Silence Costs the Room

Being right does not always repair
what being doubted publicly cost you.
Sometimes the lesson is simply
that you must be right anyway.

The patient was Margaret. Twenty-six years old. A cast on her left leg, three weeks old, from a bicycle accident that had fractured her tibia cleanly enough that the orthopedic team had not been worried about much else. She came to clinic because the leg had started to feel different. Swollen. Tighter than the cast alone should explain.

Noah examined her carefully. The calf, where he could feel it beneath the cast's edge, was warm. Tender when he pressed, in a way she had not described at her last visit. He thought about it — the hesitation of a new intern weighing a serious concern against the fear of overreacting to something ordinary.

"I want to admit her," he told Elias. "I'm worried about a DVT. The ultrasound technician had to leave to care for her child, so that won't be available until morning."

Elias looked at the chart, then at Noah. "What makes you worried," he asked — not skeptically, just carefully, the way he had learned to ask this exact question from someone who had once asked it of him.

Noah explained. "She has asymmetric swelling. The leg is warm to touch and now has tenderness that was not present at the last visit," he said.

"Admit her," Elias said. "Get the ultrasound as soon as you can in the morning."

Morning report the next day was covered by Dr. Hughes, a visiting attending standing in for someone on leave. Noah presented the case.

"Twenty-six-year-old female, leg fracture, casted, presenting with increased swelling concerning for DVT. Admitted overnight. Ultrasound pending."

Dr. Hughes laughed. Not unkindly, in his own estimation — the laugh of someone who believes he is teaching a useful lesson through humiliation.

"If we admitted every patient on the whim of an intern," he said to the room, "there wouldn't be a bed left for anyone actually sick."

A few people chuckled. Noah felt his face go warm.

Elias did not laugh. "The exam findings were suspicious," he started. Dr Hughes cut him off. "Those are typical for someone who has had a cast in place for several weeks. Any orthopedist would tell you that fact. We'll see what the ultrasound says," he said, already moving to the next case.

The ultrasound came back at noon. Extensive DVT — substantial risk for embolism, femoral and popliteal. Anticoagulation was started immediately. The admission that had drawn laughter in a room full of colleagues only a few hours earlier had very likely prevented a pulmonary embolism. Noah looked for a chance to tell those results to Dr. Hughes.

He found his chance two days later, in the hallway outside radiology.

"The ultrasound on the leg fracture patient was positive," he said. "Extensive DVT. She is on anticoagulation now."

He said it carefully — not as a confrontation, simply as information any colleague might reasonably want to know.

Dr. Hughes glanced at him. "Good outcome, then," he said, already looking past Noah toward the door, his tone carrying no weight, no acknowledgment of the room, the laughter, the dismissiveness that had preceded this entirely predictable result. "You got lucky on that one," he added, and walked on.

Noah stood in the hallway turning that sentence over.

You got lucky. Not you were right. Not I should have listened. A small deflecting phrase that let the moment close without costing Dr. Hughes anything at all.

Elias found him there a few minutes later. "You talked to him," he said. It was not quite a question.

"He said I got lucky," Noah said.

Elias was quiet. "That's probably the best you were going to get."

"Doesn't that bother you," Noah asked. "That he gets to just believe that and move on, like the room laughing at me never happened."

"It used to bother me a great deal," Elias said. "I used to think that being right should come with some kind of accounting. An apology. An acknowledgment. Something." He turned to Noah. "Mostly, it doesn't. People like Dr. Hughes will move through their careers mostly convinced of their own competence, and you will rarely get the satisfaction of watching that conviction crack in front of you."

"Then why does it matter," Noah asked, "if nobody ever has to admit they were wrong."

"Because the patient doesn't care whether Dr. Hughes apologizes," Elias said. "She cares whether the clot was found before it killed her. You weren't right so that you could be vindicated. You were right so that she could go home to her family." He paused. "The cost of being right is that it rarely feels the way you think it should. You did the work anyway. That has to be enough, most of the time, because it's usually all you're going to get."

That night Noah wrote in his notebook.

I wanted him to say I was right.
He said I got lucky instead.
The patient is alive either way.
I am going to have to learn how to let that be enough,
because the apology is not coming.

Clinical Reflection

Sometimes the diagnosis is made correctly, acted on promptly, the outcome good — and the lesson is a different one: the ordinary unfairness of being correct in a hierarchy that does not always reward correctness with acknowledgment. A senior physician's public dismissal of a junior's concern is its own form of authority bias, and when the junior turns out to be right, the senior most often faces no reckoning. No apology arrives. This is not a satisfying lesson, but it is an accurate one, and trainees deserve to hear it plainly rather than discover it, disappointed, on their own. The measure of being right is not the acknowledgment it earns you. It is the harm it prevents — and that will have to carry you through a great many rooms where the only evidence that you were right is a patient who went home.

PART III — CHAPTER 9

When the Lines Cross

Whose Patient Is She

Authority in a hospital is not a single line.
It is several lines, crossing,
and someone must know
which one holds in which room.

She had come in by helicopter the night before — a car in a multi-vehicle pileup on the interstate in heavy fog, one of several trauma cases that filled the unit that night. Multiple long bone fractures and a splenic laceration, stabilized in the OR overnight, now intubated and sedated in the surgical ICU. Elias and Noah were rounding on her along with the rest of the unit. She was improving. Vitals stable. Sedation being weaned carefully. Not yet, in Elias's reading of her, ready to come off the ventilator.

The surgery attending who had operated arrived mid-morning, moving quickly — the brisk confidence of someone with four other cases still ahead of him that day.

"Let's extubate her," he said, barely pausing at the foot of the bed. "She looks good. Get her off the vent."

Elias reviewed the chart. "She hasn't passed a spontaneous breathing trial. Her mental status is still significantly affected by the sedation we've been weaning. She's not protecting her airway reliably yet. I don't think she's ready."

The surgeon turned to him, something sharpening in his expression. "She had her surgery yesterday. I don't need a resident telling me when my patient is ready to come off the vent."

"I'm the chief resident on this unit," Elias said evenly.

"I don't care what your title is. I operated on her. She is my patient. Extubate her."

Noah stood near the door, watching — the stillness he was beginning to recognize in himself whenever a room tightened like this.

Elias did not raise his voice. "With respect," he said, "once a patient is in this unit, airway management decisions go through the ICU team. I'm not comfortable extubating her until she meets criteria."

"Comfortable," the surgeon repeated, the word carrying real impatience. "This isn't about your comfort, Resident. I have a post-op patient in recovery right now who needs an ICU bed tonight, and this one is stable enough to make room." He reached for the chart as though to write the order himself.

"I'd like to call Dr. Lighthouse," Elias said. He said it plainly — not as a threat, simply as the next correct step in a disagreement that was not going to resolve itself through repetition.

The surgeon's jaw tightened. "Fine. Call him. I have other patients." He did not leave.

Lighthouse arrived twenty minutes later. He reviewed the chart without haste, then examined the patient briefly. He turned to both of them.

"Extubating her now carries real risk — a failed extubation, reintubation under worse conditions, aspiration. She has not met the criteria we use for coming off the ventilator, and holding her was the right call." The surgeon started to speak. Lighthouse continued, without raising his voice, in a way that did not invite interruption. "In this unit, the ICU team holds final authority over ventilator management, regardless of which service performed the surgery." He looked at the surgeon directly. "That is not a courtesy. It is how this hospital keeps patients from being extubated before they are ready, by whoever is in the room with the most confidence and the least patience."

The surgeon was quiet. "She's stable," he said, his tone shifting — not quite conceding but no longer pressing forward.

"She is stable, intubated, and improving," Lighthouse said. "She will not be stable gasping for air during a failed extubation with a still-unreliable airway reflex. We will reassess this afternoon, once sedation has cleared further and she meets the criteria we actually use for this decision."

The surgeon left without another word — the silence of someone who has lost an argument he still believes, somewhere underneath the loss, he should have won.

That afternoon the patient passed her spontaneous breathing trial cleanly. Mental status clear. Extubation proceeded without complication. Had it happened that morning, on the surgeon's timeline, the outcome was far less certain.

Noah found Elias in the workroom later. "He called you Resident like it was an insult. Even though you're the chief."

"He wanted it to be one," Elias said. "It's a way of reminding someone where he thinks they belong in the room."

"Did it work," Noah asked.

"For a second," Elias said. "It always works for a second. That's exactly why you can't let the decision hinge on whether it stings. You let it sting, and you make the call anyway."

"What would have happened if Lighthouse had taken his side," Noah asked.

"Then I would have been overruled by someone with the standing to overrule me," Elias said. "That happens too, sometimes. But I still would have been right to call him, rather than just relenting in the room."

That night Noah wrote in his notebook.

Authority is not one line.
The ICU has its own. Surgery has its own.
Knowing which one holds in which room is not arrogance.
It is the only way a patient stays protected
from whoever is loudest that morning.

Clinical Reflection

The clinician pressing for speed in these collisions is rarely wrong about the goal — fewer ventilator days, earlier mobilization, a freed bed are genuine goods. The error is about timing, and about who holds the final decision in the room where the disagreement happens. One expertise governs the operation; another governs the ventilator, the sedation, the airway once the patient reaches the unit that owns them. These are different domains, each with legitimate authority inside its own boundary. When those boundaries are tested, the person with less seniority and more clarity about where the line lies is not being insubordinate by holding it. Know the line. Hold it, even when someone louder insists it doesn't exist.

PART III — CHAPTER 10

What the Bed Conceals

The View from the Chair

The bed is not a neutral surface.
It conceals as much as it supports.
What a patient looks like lying still
is not always what he looks like
when asked to live upright.

The patient was two days post-op from coronary artery bypass surgery.

Noah had rounded on him that morning. Checked the incision. Reviewed the overnight vitals. Listened to the lungs — diminished at the bases, expected. Palpated the pedal pulses. Documented them as present, faint bilaterally, consistent with the mild peripheral vascular disease already noted in the surgical summary. He had been in the room for twelve minutes. The patient had been supine for all of them.

That was the problem. Not the twelve minutes. The supine.

Sandra Reed had been a nurse on the cardiothoracic step-down unit for nineteen years.

She got him up at two in the afternoon — standard protocol, day two post-CABG, early mobilization to prevent atelectasis and reduce the risk of DVT. She helped him pivot to the edge of the bed. Got his feet onto the floor. Walked him the three steps to the chair beside the window and helped him settle.

Then she looked down.

His left leg, from the knee downward, had gone blue. Not the mild mottling of dependent edema or venous pooling. Blue. A color that did not belong in a living limb. Mottled at the foot, darker toward the ankle — the discoloration of tissue not receiving what it needs.

She had seen enough post-surgical complications in nineteen years to know she was not imagining it.

She did not move him back to bed. She paged Noah immediately.

Noah arrived four minutes later. He studied the leg. Then he looked at Sandra.

"How long has it been like this," he said.

"Since I sat him up," she said. "It wasn't there when he was in bed. I checked him at noon. Both legs looked the same."

Noah examined the leg carefully. The left foot was cool — cooler than the right by a degree that was not subtle. The dorsalis pedis pulse, present this morning, was now absent. The posterior tibial, also absent. The patient described a heaviness in the leg, a pressure he hadn't had before.

"Did it hurt when you stood," Noah asked.

The man nodded. "Figured it was just stiff. From lying down so long."

Noah watched Sandra. "Good catch," he said. He was already reaching for his pager.

He found Elias in the workroom.

"Post-CABG, day two. Sixty-eight-year-old. Left leg goes blue when he sits up. Disappears when he's supine. Absent pulses at the foot. Present this morning on rounds."

Elias looked up. "Position-dependent," he said.

"Yes."

Elias was already standing. "There's an embolus in his leg. Probably occurred during the surgery — or when he came off bypass. It obstructs the artery just enough to be visible only when the leg is dependent. Supine, he still gets enough flow that you don't see it. Have you paged Vascular?"

"Already done, and they're on the way," Noah said.

The vascular surgery fellow arrived within ten minutes. The assessment was rapid. Acute limb ischemia, early — caught, the vascular attending said, at a point where intervention was still straightforward. Had it gone unrecognized through the night, the ischemic leg would have been compromised and the surgery much more complicated.

The patient was taken back to the OR that afternoon. Embolectomy. The clot retrieved cleanly. Perfusion restored.

That evening Noah found Sandra at the nursing station.

"I wanted to come back and tell you how it went," he said. "They got it. He's going to keep the leg."

She looked up. "Good," she said. It was not a small word the way she said it.

"You saved it," Noah said. "I examined him this morning. Supine. I checked his pulses, documented them, moved on. I had no idea."

"You checked what was there to check," she said. "I just happened to be the one who got him out of bed."

"That's the point, though," Noah said. "You were the one who got him out of bed. And you knew what you were looking at when you saw it."

She was quiet a beat. "Nineteen years," she said. "You see things."

"But you knew there was more to it. That is what matters," said Noah.

Noah found Elias afterward.

"She didn't call me because she was certain," Noah said. "She called me because she was concerned. She saw something that looked wrong and she didn't talk herself out of it."

"What would you have done," Elias said, "if she had called and said — I sat him up and his leg looks a little blue, is that normal."

Noah thought about it. "I'd like to think I would have come."

"Would you have," Elias said. Not critically. Carefully.

Noah was honest. "I don't know," he said. "It's day two post-CABG. There are a lot of patients."

"She didn't ask you a question," Elias said. "She paged you like it was a problem. That's why you came immediately. That's a skill. Not every nurse uses it. Not every physician responds to it the way you did." He paused. "The finding was position dependent. You could not have seen it from the position you examine patients in. She saw it because she was the one who changed his position. That's not luck. That's what she does all day, in ways the chart doesn't fully capture."

He turned to Noah. "She paged you without hesitation. She knew you would come. That means something. Don't forget it."

That night Noah wrote in his notebook.

I examined him supine. She examined him upright.
We were looking at the same patient.
We were not looking at the same leg.
She knew what she was looking at.
She knew I would come.
Both of those things mattered.

Clinical Reflection

Some findings cannot be seen from where physicians usually stand. A patient examined flat, for a few minutes on rounds, presents only the version that position allows; what is invisible supine may be obvious upright — and the person present when the patient sits up is usually not the physician. This is the quiet asymmetry of who observes whom: physicians see patients in fixed postures, briefly, on a schedule, while nurses turn them, sit them up, and stay through the hours when a finding first declares itself. Which places a burden on the physician that has nothing to do with knowledge. Build the kind of presence that makes the people who spend those hours feel it is worth the trouble to tell you — and notice how they tell you. A concern raised as a question can be set aside; the same concern stated as a finding demands a response.

PART III — CHAPTER 11

The Discovery

The Teacher Becomes the Patient

The method does not care who you are.
It asks the same questions of everyone.
Even the person who taught it.

It began with his vision. A curtain, he would describe it later, drawing across the left eye from the side, lasting perhaps thirty seconds, then lifting as cleanly as it had arrived. Lighthouse sat at his desk and waited for it to pass. It passed. He noted the time.

The slurring began four minutes later. He was dictating a note when he heard it in his own voice — a softness to certain consonants, an imprecision that had not been there a moment before. He stopped dictating. He stood. He walked to the small mirror hung near the door of his office and looked at his face. The left side was not quite right. A subtle asymmetry, the kind a stranger might not notice, that a clinician could not miss.

He did not call 911. He called Elias.

"I need you to come to the ER," he said. "I'm coming in now. I want you to admit me."

A pause on the line.

"Are you all right," Elias said.

"I had a transient visual disturbance. Left eye. And some dysarthria. It's resolving. But I need to be seen, and I want someone I trust to do it."

He walked. His office was in the building adjacent, connected by a covered corridor he had crossed thousands of times. The symptoms had passed by then. His gait was steady. He knew, even so, that a physician who has just had a TIA should not be walking anywhere alone. He walked anyway. Lighthouse had spent a lengthy career making careful distinctions between what he would advise and what he would do himself, and he had never entirely reconciled the gap between them.

Elias met him at the door. It was the first time in all the years they had worked together that Elias had seen him as a patient — Lighthouse walking through those doors in street clothes, without his white coat, without the authority that had always preceded him into every room. It required a moment to absorb.

"Tell me what happened," Elias said. He said it the way Lighthouse had once taught him — calmly, without rushing, making room for the whole story.

Lighthouse told it precisely. The visual curtain. The duration. The dysarthria. The mirror. The timeline. Elias listened without interrupting. When Lighthouse finished, Elias said, "I need to do an exam."

The neurological exam was largely normal by the time it was performed; the deficits having cleared — consistent with a transient event rather than a completed stroke. The MRI showed no infarct. The carotid ultrasound showed no significant stenosis. The EKG showed normal sinus rhythm. Everything pointed toward a cryptogenic TIA — a transient ischemic attack without an immediately obvious source, the kind of event that, in a man of Lighthouse's age, demanded a thorough search for an explanation that basic workup had not yet provided.

Elias stood at the nursing station after reviewing the results, the differential narrowing in his mind. One possibility kept returning. He did not say it aloud. He ordered the echocardiogram — and left the bubble study off it, the very thing he suspected, and went back to the room and said nothing. He wanted to see the workup through the way Lighthouse had always taught him — without closing the question before the room had a chance to find it.

Maya arrived mid-morning, having heard from Elias. She stood in the doorway, looking at Lighthouse in the bed.

"I'm all right," Lighthouse said, before she could speak.

"You had a TIA," she said.

"I did. Elias is working it up properly."

She nodded. She pulled up a chair and opened the chart on the tablet in her hand. She read quietly.

"Have you had an echocardiogram yet," she asked.

"Scheduled for this afternoon," Elias said from across the room. There was no urgency in his voice. He had learned, over years, how to wait without showing it.

Maya studied the chart a moment longer. "We need to add a bubble study," she said, and reached over and put it on the order Elias had written.

Something passed between Elias and Lighthouse — brief, almost imperceptible. The acknowledgment of two people who had already arrived at the same place and had been waiting, without saying so, to see if someone else would get there first. They had not needed to wait long.

"Walk me through your thinking," Elias said.

"No carotid disease, no atrial fibrillation, no source anyone had found." Maya set the tablet down. "Which leaves the thing you only find if you look for it — a PFO. A clot from the venous side traverses it and reaches the brain instead of being filtered out by the lungs. The bubble study is how you catch it." She looked at Lighthouse. "It's worth asking."

Lighthouse watched her. "Yes," he said. He glanced at Elias. "It is."

Noah arrived that afternoon. He stood in the hallway, uncertain whether to go in. Elias found him there.

"He wants you in there," Elias said. "He asked for all of you."

The study was done that afternoon in the echo lab. The cardiologist was one Elias had called personally — someone he trusted, someone who would take care with this patient without needing to be told why. The agitated saline went in. They watched the screen together — Elias, Maya, Noah, the cardiologist, and Lighthouse himself, who had asked to watch and did so with the focused attention of a man who has spent a career reading clinical data and has not stopped simply because he is now its source.

The bubbles filled the right atrium first — a bright, immediate cloud of them, exactly where they belonged. Then, three beats later, they appeared in the left atrium, where no bubble should ever be unless there is an opening between the two chambers. The shunt was real.

"There it is," Maya said.

Nobody else spoke.

Patent foramen ovale — a small flap between the heart's two upper chambers, open in everyone before birth and, in about one adult in four, never fully sealed. In him it had stayed silent for six decades, until a clot found its way through it and traveled to his brain.

There was still the question of where the clot had come from. Elias ordered an ultrasound of both legs, searching for a deep-vein clot that might have been its source — the kind of origin that, in these cases, is found less often than not. He added a cardiac monitor as well, to watch the coming days for a brief run of atrial fibrillation, too short to have surfaced on a single tracing. The PFO explained how a clot could reach the brain. It did not, by itself, explain where the clot had begun.

The cardiologist outlined the options. Medical management. Anticoagulation. Or percutaneous closure — a catheter-based procedure that could seal the PFO without open surgery. Lighthouse listened carefully, asked precise questions, and was, Elias thought watching him, the same person he had always been in a clinical conversation. Methodical. Unhurried. Interested in the full picture before he formed a view. Only the white coat was missing.

Later, after the cardiologist had left and the room had grown quieter, Lighthouse looked at the three of them — Elias, Maya, Noah — sitting in the arrangement of people who do not want to leave a room where something important has just happened.

"Maya," he said. She turned to him. "The bubble study. What made you think of it."

"The workup kept coming back without an answer," she said. "I asked myself what would make this not what we'd already found." She paused. "I think I've been asking that question long enough that I don't always notice when I'm asking it."

Lighthouse nodded slowly. "No," he said. "You probably don't." He was quiet. "That is exactly what it looks like when something has actually been learned."

He looked at Noah. "When Maya suggested the bubble study — what did you think."

"I thought she was right," Noah said. "The source hadn't been found. It was the next question to ask."

"Did you know about PFO and cryptogenic TIA before today."

"I knew about it," Noah said. "I don't know if I would have thought of it myself, in this room, today."

"That's honest," Lighthouse said. "Knowing something and reaching for it at the right moment are different skills. The second one takes longer."

He studied Elias last. Elias, who had admitted him. Who had taken his history the way he had been taught. Who had ordered the echocardiogram, left the bubble study off it on purpose, and then stood back and let Maya be the one to add it.

"You let her lead," Lighthouse said.

"She saw it first," Elias said.

"You made room for her to," Lighthouse said. "That is not the same thing as waiting."

Elias didn't answer. Lighthouse looked at him a while longer. He had made Elias chief resident at the start of the year — one of the youngest he had ever named in his years as Chief of Medicine, young enough that he had wondered, even then, whether he was right to do it. He had made the same kind of early call once, with a resident named Mann, and had spent a long time afterward unsure. In a few months Elias would leave for a fellowship in critical care. Watching him now — standing back, letting the room find its own way to the answer — Lighthouse thought the decision had been the right one.

"I have spent a long time teaching people to ask better questions than they would have asked without me," he said. "I did not expect to be the patient who would need them to." He looked at the three of them. "Thank you," he said.

That night, in separate places, three people wrote in their notebooks.

Maya wrote:

He asked what made me think of it.
I told him the truth: I've been asking that question long enough that I don't always notice.
I think that might be the only real measure
of whether a habit has taken hold.

Noah wrote:

I knew about PFO.
I don't know if I would have thought of it today.
The gap between knowing and reaching is where
the next few years of my training live.

Elias wrote:

I let her lead.
He said that is not the same thing as waiting.
I am still thinking about the difference.

Clinical Reflection

There is a difference between making room for someone and waiting for them, and it is not always visible from outside. The senior reaches the answer first and says nothing — not to withhold it, but because a question supplied from above proves only that the teacher is still teaching, while a question that arrives on its own proves it has been learned. He orders the study and lets the room come to it. That is the last examination a teacher gives, and the student rarely knows it is being administered. A habit that works only while its author is in the room was never truly passed on. This one had outlived the need for him before he ever lay down in the bed.

PART III — CHAPTER 12

The Habit That Outlives the Room

What Remains

Teaching ends when the habit no longer requires the teacher.
What is left is not a method.
It is a way of standing at the bedside
when the answer has not yet arrived.

The patient was thirty-eight years old. She had been seen three times in the past six weeks. Once in urgent care. Once in the emergency department. Once by her primary care physician, who had referred her here with a note that read, simply: Something is wrong. I don't know what.

Noah picked up her chart on a Tuesday morning — the kind of morning that does not announce itself as significant. He read the prior notes carefully. Fever, recurring, spiking in the afternoons and resolving by morning, the rhythm that made each individual encounter seem less alarming than the pattern of them together. Joint pain, fluctuating — wrists, knees, ankles, moving between them without settling anywhere long enough to be definitively examined in its worst state. Labs mildly abnormal. Elevated inflammatory markers. White count slightly up. Nothing that by itself demanded a name.

He presented her on rounds the way he had learned to present — completely, without editing toward a conclusion he hadn't yet reached. He laid out the pieces. The fever pattern. The migratory arthralgia. The elevated markers. He did not name a diagnosis.

"I don't know yet what this is," he said. "But I think these pieces belong to the same thing."

Maya had seen the patient the evening before, covering a late admission. She added one thing.

"Every prior note says no rash," Maya said. "When I saw her last night she told me the same — no rash, she'd have remembered one." She paused. "So this morning, before rounds, I went back and asked it a different way. Not whether she'd had a rash — whether her skin ever changed. That she remembered. It comes up across her chest and arms in the afternoons, when the fever climbs, and it's gone before anyone comes to look. Faint, blotchy. She never called it a rash, because to her it wasn't one." Maya paused. "The color she described was salmon — that pale pink of a salmon fillet in the market case."

The room was quiet.

Elias raised an eyebrow. "Fever. Migratory arthritis. An evanescent salmon rash no one has ever caught, because it fades before anyone thinks to ask," he said. He did not say the diagnosis. He let the room hold it.

Noah felt it forming.

"What else do we need," Elias asked.

"Labs," Noah said slowly. "Something that confirms systemic inflammation at this degree." He paused. "Ferritin."

Elias watched him. "Has anyone checked a ferritin."

Nobody had.

The result came back that afternoon. Markedly elevated — more than twenty times the upper limit of normal, the degree of elevation that, in this clinical context, was not simply a marker of inflammation but a signature of it. The laboratory finding that transformed a constellation of individually nonspecific symptoms into something nameable.

Adult-onset Still's disease.

That afternoon Noah was at the bedside reviewing the result with the patient when she said, almost as an aside: "It's happening again. The skin thing."

Noah looked. Across her upper chest and arms, faint at first, then more visible — a salmon-colored eruption, macular, evanescent even as he watched it, beginning to fade at its edges while its center still declared itself. He did not reach for his phone. He stood and looked, the way he had been taught to look, carefully and without rushing, for as long as the finding was willing to be seen. It lasted perhaps four minutes. Then it was gone.

He wrote in the chart: Evanescent salmon-colored rash observed directly, upper chest and bilateral arms, duration approximately four minutes, consistent with clinical diagnosis.

Rheumatology was consulted. They confirmed the diagnosis within the hour; the clinical picture now complete enough that the pattern was unmistakable. Treatment was begun.

The patient asked what the diagnosis meant. Noah explained it carefully — what it was, what it wasn't, what treatment looked like, what she could expect. He sat down while he explained it. He did not rush. He asked, at the end, whether she had questions. She had several. He answered each one.

Lighthouse arrived late that afternoon. He had not been part of the morning. Had not been called. He read the chart. Reviewed the ferritin result. Did not say anything. Then he went to find Noah.

Noah was at the bedside. Not examining. Not charting. Simply sitting — the way he had been taught, by people who had been taught by someone else, that sitting was itself a clinical act, sometimes the most important one. The patient was talking. Something about her children, about how long this had been going on, about how relieved she was to finally have a name for it. Noah was listening. Not performing listening. Not waiting for the next clinical data point. Listening the way a person listens when they are genuinely present in a room with another person, without anywhere else they need to be.

Lighthouse stood in the doorway. He watched, then stepped back into the hallway.

Elias found him there.

"You're not going in," Elias said.

"No," Lighthouse said. He was quiet. "He doesn't need me in there."

It was not said with pride exactly. It was said the way someone states a fact they have been waiting a long time to be able to state.

They stood together in the hallway, the two of them, listening to the faint sound of a conversation continuing on the other side of the door. Neither of them spoke. There was nothing left that needed to be said in the hallway. The work, for now, was happening in the room.

Clinical Reflection

The clinician who learns to ask the key question does not remember where they learned it. The question that unlocks the diagnosis is reached without prompting — the way language becomes natural. Once the habit is engrained, it is simply present, without needing its originator to be named. The room is empty now, and the people who modeled it for you are no longer there. But the question — and the modeling of it — is still being asked, in new rooms, by new people who will model it for others without recalling where they first learned it. That is the only kind of teaching that lasts.

Afterword

The book ends in a doorway, and that was deliberate.

Lighthouse does not enter the room, because he is no longer needed in it. That is the only honest measure of teaching there is. Not the evaluations, not the gratitude, not the lecture that went well. Whether the habit survives your absence. You do not get to know while you are still teaching. You find out standing in a hallway, listening to a conversation you are not part of, hearing your own question asked by someone who no longer remembers where they learned it.

If you are a student or a resident, I want to tell you plainly what I could not have heard at your stage: the notebook matters. Not the notes about doses and criteria — those are in your pocket already, on a device that knows more than I ever did. The other notebook. The one where you write down what a case cost you, what you almost missed, what you decided at two in the morning and why. Every learner in this book keeps one. That was not a literary device. The clinicians I most admired all kept some version of it, and the act of writing the lesson in your own words, on the night it happened, is what converts an experience into a habit. Experience alone does not teach. Examined experience does.

If you have been practicing for many years, some of these chapters will have been uncomfortable, and one or two of them may have been personal. Most physicians who practice long enough, and honestly enough, carry a small number of patients where something they did, or did not do, or deferred to someone else, changed how the story ended. I carry mine. Lighthouse says in these pages that pretending the list does not exist is its own kind of harm, and I wrote that sentence for myself before I gave it to him. The list is not a private failure. It is a shared condition of doing this work honestly, and the only thing it asks of us is that we let it make us better at the bedside rather than more defended away from it.

And if you are not in medicine at all — if you came to this book as a patient, or as someone who loves one — then you have seen, from the inside, why the woman lying flat on the table matters, why the man who says this pain is different deserves to be heard the first time he says it, and why the question a clinician asks from a chair is worth more than the ten asked from the doorway. You are allowed to say the thing that does not fit. You are allowed to say it twice. The good ones are listening for it.

A fair question hangs over a book about medical error written in this decade: does every chapter argue for handing the work to artificial intelligence sooner. Some of it, honestly, yes. A machine reading the whole record would have flagged a potassium that climbed across four admissions while everyone called it baseline. It would have connected a port-a-cath documented in four notes to the swollen face sitting directly above it. It would have seen two sisters with the same failing kidneys on two different floors without needing the accident of one resident covering both. Pattern across time and across charts is exactly what these systems do not get tired of. And a robotic surgeon will never arrive at midnight smelling of alcohol — though I notice the question does not die there. Will it operate with a failing part it believes it can compensate for. Overconfidence, it turns out, may not be an exclusively human disease.

But look at where the diagnoses in this book actually came from. A wife's aside about a dog that wouldn't eat. A dying preacher's request that made no sense by the numbers. A woman who confessed something she had never told her husband, only after a resident sat still long enough to be worth telling. It was a physician in Flint, Dr. Mona Hanna-Attisha, working from the same electronic records everyone else had, who saw what the lead was doing to the children — the data was there for anyone; she decided it mattered, and said so out loud, at professional risk, until someone listened. The most important findings in these pages arrived through trust, and trust is extended to someone, not something. I am not certain patients will hand their secrets to a machine that remembers everything and answers to whom, exactly.

So, my wager, for the visible arc of the future, is on the human in the room — a clinician using these tools the way Lighthouse used a stethoscope, as an extension of attention rather than a replacement for it. The machine will catch what the tired mind misses. The human will hear what the machine was never told. A physician with both will be better than either alone. The moment this book is about — a diagnosis feels settled, and someone decides whether to stop — will still belong to whoever is standing at the bedside. I hope they are wise enough to bring the machine with them, and wiser still about which of them should widen the lens. Then teach it to someone, without telling them you are teaching it — and one day, stand in the doorway and find out whether it took.

A personal note. My mother died of non-Hodgkin's lymphoma in 1985, during my residency — not medical school, as it is for Elias in this book. The story of her saying "Daddy" is entirely true. Her cancer is now among modern medicine's quiet miracles, a disease whose treatment offers real hope of a cure. She did not live long enough to see me become the physician, husband, and father I grew into. I hope she would have been proud of me.

W.H.L.

William H. Light, M.D., practiced internal medicine for nearly forty years and served as chief resident in 1985. He has spent his career teaching the way he believes medicine is best learned — through attention, modeled judgment, and the steady habits that keep patients safe. The Lighthouse Principle is the first book in a series on the quiet craft of clinical reasoning.

ALSO BY WILLIAM H. LIGHT, M.D.

Outlast: Your Budget Friendly Guide to Life Extension

Outlast II: A Physician's Longevity Guide for the Generation That Cannot Wait (forthcoming)

THE LIGHTHOUSE PRINCIPLE Series

The Lighthouse Principle

The Machine in the Room (forthcoming)

The Making of a Clinician (forthcoming)

www.ingramcontent.com/pod-product-compliance
Lightning Source LLC
LaVergne TN
LVHW010720061126
851857LV00014B/1270
9798997163211